PROSPECTIVE
LONGEVITY

PROSPECTIVE LONGEVITY

A New Vision of Population Aging

WARREN C. SANDERSON AND SERGEI SCHERBOV

Harvard University Press

Cambridge, Massachusetts
London, England
2019

Library of Congress Cataloging-in-Publication Data

Names: Sanderson, Warren C., author. | Scherbov, Sergei, author.
Title: Prospective longevity : a new vision of population aging /
Warren C. Sanderson and Sergei Scherbov.
Description: Cambridge, Massachusetts : Harvard University Press, 2019. |
Includes bibliographical references and index.
Identifiers: LCCN 2019014642 | ISBN 9780674975613
Subjects: LCSH: Population aging—Statistical methods. | Ability, Influence
of age on. | Biometry. | Longevity.
Classification: LCC HQ1061 .S3117 2019 | DDC 304.6/1—dc23
LC record available at https://lccn.loc.gov/2019014642

CONTENTS

PROSPECTIVE
LONGEVITY

Introduction

The Importance of Clear Vision

If you were hiking one day and you encountered a mountain lion, what would you do? The advice given to people is to raise your arms to appear as large as possible, make noise, and act unafraid. But if your vision were highly distorted and what you were really seeing was a pet cat, you might become agitated as it came toward you, but you would certainly be chagrined when it brushed your leg asking to be petted. Other people watching you, your arm motions, your screaming, and your attempt to act unafraid as the cat approached you, might wonder about the appropriateness of your actions.

If you were hiking one day and saw a small tree branch lying on the ground, you might be tempted to step on it in order to experience the satisfying sound of the branch snapping in two. But if your vision were highly distorted, and what was lying on your path was really a rattlesnake, you would hear instead a less satisfying sound, one that could lead to undesirable effects on your well-being.

Whenever possible, it is desirable to help people distinguish between mountain lions and pet cats, and between downed tree branches and rattlesnakes. It is desirable to see more clearly what is in front of us so that we can take appropriate actions. In the field of population aging, our vision has been highly distorted. The goal of this book is to correct those distortions and provide a clearer vision. It is to keep us from screaming when there is nothing to scream at and to keep us safe as we go forward.

Population aging is a complex, multidimensional phenomenon. We encounter many such phenomena in our everyday life. Weather is one of these. When we walk outside, we get a feeling of how warm it is, how humid it is, and how hard the wind is blowing, among other things, but we cannot see the temperature, the humidity, and the wind speed with the naked eye. To see what the temperature, humidity, and wind speed are, we use instruments to measure them: thermometers for temperature, hygrometers for humidity, and anemometers for wind speed. Scientific studies of weather patterns are based on detailed measurements made with those instruments. Population aging is similar. We can walk outside and see how old people look and talk to people about how old they feel, but systematic studies of population aging require detailed measurements. Unfortunately, most measurements of population aging that we have had up to now do not allow us to see very clearly. It is like having thermometers that showed the same reading when the temperature was 32 degrees Fahrenheit (0 degree Celsius) and when it was 50 degrees Fahrenheit (10 degrees Celsius). Although, in the past, the older instruments did help us see population aging better, it is now clear that there is a great deal that they did not allow us to see. It was like wearing a pair of glasses that improved our vision a bit but still were not strong enough to allow us to read. The purpose of this book is to provide you with a new set of glasses, one that provides you with the ability to see the multiple dimensions of population aging more clearly. After you walk around the demographic environment with your new glasses on, we think that you will never want to take them off.

How We Look at Population Aging

At its most fundamental level, the choice of which glasses to use depends on one's conceptualization of age itself. Our view of age is akin to the World Health Organization's (WHO). In their report *World Report of Ageing and Health* (WHO 2015), aging is conceptualized on the basis of "functional ability," not chronological age.

"Functional ability comprises the health-related attributes that enable people to be and to do what they have reason to value. It is made up of the intrinsic capacity of the individual, relevant environmental characteristics and the interactions between the individual and these characteristics" (28).

"As the evidence shows, the loss of ability typically associated with ageing is only loosely related to a person's chronological age" (vii).

Our view of age is similar, but what we choose to look at is different. The WHO views aging from the perspective of the functional ability of individuals. We view aging from a population perspective and analyze it in terms of characteristics of populations related to functional ability, such as remaining life expectancy and freedom from disabilities.

What Do Statistical Agencies See?

The changing functional abilities of older people are visible everywhere except in what most major statistical agencies tell us. Those agencies produce tables and graphs based on the premise that people of some fixed age are functionally equivalent in terms of population aging regardless of where or when they lived.

For example, for many years, the United Nations put everyone 60 and over in the category of "older persons." An early United Nations' document on aging was the *Vienna International Plan of Action on Aging* (1983), which stated,

> Only in the past few decades has the attention of national societies and the world community been drawn to the social, economic, political and scientific questions raised by the phenomenon of aging on a massive scale. In 1950, according to United Nations estimates, there were approximately 200 million persons 60 years of age and over throughout the world. By 1975, their number had increased to 350 million. United Nations projections to the year 2000 indicate that the number will increase to 590 million, and by the year 2025 to over 1,100 million; that is, an increase of 224 per cent since 1975 (United Nations 1983).

Over 3 decades later, in the United Nations' *World Population Ageing 2015*, we have

> According to data from World Population Prospects: the 2015 Revision (United Nations, 2015), the number of older persons—those aged

60 years or over—has increased substantially in recent years in most countries and regions, and that growth is projected to accelerate in the coming decades.

Between 2015 and 2030, the number of people in the world aged 60 years or over is projected to grow by 56 per cent, from 901 million to 1.4 billion, and by 2050, the global population of older persons is projected to more than double its size in 2015, reaching nearly 2.1 billion. (United Nations 2015, 1–2)

Those passages were written using the old pair of glasses, where 60-year-olds in 1982 looked just as old as 60-year-olds in 2015. To other agencies—including Eurostat (2017), the official statistical agency of the European Union, the US Census Bureau (He et al. 2016), and the Organisation for Economic Co-operation and Development (OECD 2016)—all 65-year-olds looked identical. It is as if all of them were wearing glasses through which they could not see the differing characteristics of people.

There are many reasons why so many organizations would produce the same sorts of numbers. First, measures of aging have been based on data which show the number of people in a population at each age. These data come from censuses, surveys, or estimates. They immediately show the numbers of people above age 60 or 65, so no additional information is needed. Second, the proportions of people 60+ or 65+ in a country are immediately standardized. It is not necessary to compute different ages for different countries or time periods. The third reason is that these figures produce historically consistent and comparable time series.

The conventional figures on population aging have been produced and discussed for well over half a century and, up to now, there has been no accepted alternative. After all, to be an improvement on the conventional measures, any alternatives would also have to be easy to compute, readily standardized, and produce historically consistent time series. We have been publishing in the field for well over a decade and have produced an accepted alternative. In *World Population Ageing 2017*, the United Nations (2017a) has now accepted one of our measures of population aging and included it along with more conventional ones.

Although like all academics, we always wish that people would immediately accept our work, this is neither how the world works nor how it should. New ideas must be tested before they are accepted. The ideas must be around long enough for people to get to know them inside and out. Thorough testing of new ideas is particularly important for the United Nations Population Division, whose figures on population aging are the de facto world standard. But now there are 2 sets of eyeglasses. With the old set, wearers were blind to any other feature of people except their chronological ages. With ours, many previously unobservable characteristics of people become visible. The fact that the United Nations has accepted one of our measures certainly does not mean it has accepted the rest of what is written in this book. It takes a while to get used to a new set of glasses.

The Necessity of Choice

Is it worthwhile even trying on the new glasses? After all, the old ones have been serviceable for many years. Nevertheless, the vision when wearing them has never been very clear. This is immediately observable when using data on life expectancy. The United Nations has made estimates of life expectancy for 5-year intervals from 1950–1955 to 2010–2015 and forecasts onward to 2095–2100. According to the United Nations figures, 65-year-old Chinese women in 1950–1955 had a remaining life expectancy of 8.72 years and 65-year-old Japanese women in 2095–2100 are forecasted to have a remaining life expectancy of 29.80 years. Wearing the old glasses, people could only see that these women were 65 years old. Nothing else about them would be visible. For over a decade, we have been writing about population aging from a new perspective, one that takes into account the changing characteristics of people. With the new glasses, many differences between those Chinese and Japanese women are now observable.

In the study of population aging, does it matter which glasses are worn? It is simple to answer this question. The United Nations' website (United Nations 2017f) makes it easy to try on the new glasses. Here's an example of the differences in what can be seen. Using the old glasses, it appears that the population of northern Europe grew older between 1980 and 2015. Using the new glasses, it can be seen that it grew younger. We show in this book that one's vision of population

aging is very different depending on whether the changing characteristics of people are considered or not.

Adjusting to the New Glasses

We argue here that our new measures of population aging enable us to
see past and possible future patterns of population aging more clearly.
But before we recommend their use, we have to discuss whether there
are any disadvantages of doing so. Up to now, there have been three
main disadvantages of using our measures. The most important is the
cost associated with deviating from what the United Nations published. One aspect of this is the difficulty that nonexperts have of
evaluating our new measures. Nonexperts generally had no way of assessing whether our new measures make sense and, if so, how to use
them. Even if nonexperts had made the effort of learning about our
measures of population aging, they would have found few people to
talk with about them.

Now that *World Population Ageing 2017* presents readers with a
choice of measures, the assessment of the costs and benefits of understanding our new measures changes. First, the United Nations now ac-
cepts one of our measures, so, when using it, there is no longer any
cost to deviating from what the United Nations publishes. Second,
people now have an incentive to learn about our measures, because
they know that other people will be doing so as well. So, what was, for
many people, an almost insurmountable barrier to the use of our measures of aging has now vanished.

The second problem faced by potential users of our measures of
aging was that they often did not know where to find them. Now,
however, one of them is published in *World Population Ageing 2017*
along with all the other measures of aging users are familiar with. Our
new measures of population aging can also be found on our website,
www.reaging.org. So, the problem of finding our new measures has
also vanished.

A further difficulty remains. The conventional measures often categorize people as being old starting at age 65. With our new set of glasses,
things look different and it might take a while for people's vision to
adjust.

The Demographic Landscape

In this book, we travel through the demographic landscape looking at its interesting features at first through conventional lenses and then through the new ones that we describe here. With the new glasses, it is as though we are in a different place, everything looks so different. We hike on the path where the mountain lion was perceived, but we see only a house cat and we are careful not to step on any rattlesnakes.

The data that we use are all publicly available and all our analyses are replicable. The data that we use most frequently have been published by the United Nations. We use two sorts of United Nations data, population distributions by age and sex, and mortality rate data organized in what are called life tables. The United Nations has produced age distributions for each of its countries and for some related regions at 5-year intervals from 1950 to 2015 and made forecasts of them to 2100. This was an incredibly difficult task, because for many countries and dates there were just fragments of data or none at all. The United Nations has also produced corresponding life tables, which are sets of organized data derived from age-specific mortality rates. They tell us the life expectancy at each age and allow us to compute statistics like 5-year survival rates at each age. The United Nations life tables are used in forecasting population age structures, and, therefore, the United Nations age structures and life tables are consistent with one another.

United Nations life tables are produced for 5-year intervals. Estimates are made for the periods 1950–1955 to 2010–2015 and forecasts are made for 2015–2020 to 2095–2100. In Japan, for example, life expectancy at age 65 (both sexes combined) was 12.51 years in 1950–1955 and the United Nations forecasts it to be 29.90 years in 2095–2100. We rely heavily on United Nations age structures and life tables in this book. They are so easily available on the United Nations website with a few clicks of the mouse that it is easy to forget how remarkable they really are. We also often use life tables from the Human Mortality Database (HMD) (University of California, Berkeley, and Max Planck Institute for Demographic Research 2017). In terms of data, the demographic environment is much richer now than it was when the conventional measures of population aging first appeared. The old glasses sufficed in an environment in which there was little to see in the first place. But it would be a shame to continue wearing them today.

A New View

Aging is a multidimensional phenomenon. This book presents a new vision of how population aging should be conceptualized and measured. Our contribution is in quantifying aspects of population aging, taking the differing characteristics of populations into account. So, we have called our methodology the "characteristics approach" to the study of population aging. The characteristics approach allows us to see aspects of population aging that were not visible before and this has required that we produce names for those new things. To avoid confusion, the first time that we encounter those names and other technical terms in each chapter, we put them in italics. It is important to note that the italicized terms have specific technical definitions. A glossary containing those definitions can be found following the conclusion.

This book is best read in order. Later chapters often make use of ideas developed in the earlier ones. Most chapters have a dual purpose: to describe a new methodology for quantifying aspects of population aging and to implement that methodology. Chapter 1 focuses on the old pair of glasses and provides a history of some of the measures of population aging that are still in use. One measure is the *total dependency ratio (TDR)*, defined generally as the ratio of those categorized as dependents to those who are not. To our knowledge, the first TDR appeared in German in a book by Carl Ballod (1913). The old glasses, then, are over a century old. While there have been major changes in data availability and the computing environment, the old glasses remain, more or less, what they were in 1913.

In Chapter 2, we put on the new pair of eyeglasses. When people are young, it makes sense to think of people in terms of their chronological ages. The World Health Organization has standards for what 1-year-old children should look like, what 2-year-old children should look like, and onward through age 5. These standards are based on chronological age. They include length/height-for-age; weight-for-age; weight-for-length/height; body mass index-for-age; head circumference-for-age; arm circumference-for-age; subscapular skinfold-for-age; triceps skinfold-for-age; motor development milestones; weight velocity; length velocity; and head circumference velocity (WHO 2017b). The WHO maintains that those standards "can be applied to all children everywhere, regardless of ethnicity, socioeconomic status and type of feeding" (WHO 2017a).

For older people, who have aged at different rates, chronological age is much less informative. There are no universal standards for how a 71-year-old, for example, should become a 72-year-old. The level of health, disability, and cognition for older people are more closely related to how much longer they have to live than how long they have already lived. So, in Chapter 2, we see age as two-dimensional. People have both a chronological age and a *prospective age.* People who share the same chronological age have lived the same number of years. However, people who share the same prospective age are in age groups where they have the same remaining life expectancy. The calculation of prospective age is similar to the calculation that economists make when they take inflation into account. Economists normally adjust quantities for inflation using price indexes. Prospective ages are similar to inflation adjusted quantities, except that they use life tables instead of price indexes. Informally, prospective age can be thought of as an adjustment for "age inflation" caused by changes in longevity.

Putting on a new pair of glasses can be disorienting at first and that may be your experience. At first, it looks like we are seeing double, and, indeed, we are. We are used to people having only one age. Now, people have two, a backward-looking chronological age and a forward-looking prospective age. It is a giant step from wearing glasses that only allow us to see things in one dimension (chronological age) to glasses that allow us to see things in two dimensions (chronological age and prospective age).

In Chapter 3, we ask the question, How old do you need to be to be "old"? It may seem like an odd question at first, but we are no longer in a one-dimensional world. In the one-dimensional world, everyone is categorized as "old" or perhaps an "old-age dependent" at some fixed chronological age, usually 60 or 65. It does not matter when the person lived, where the person lived or anything else about the person. The one-dimensional world view required just one number for everyone everywhere and always.

In the two-dimensional world, the question of the age at which people are categorized as old becomes more interesting. In our previous papers and in this book, we categorize people as old when they are approaching the ends of their lives. We make this concrete by categorizing people as old when they are in age groups where their remaining life expectancy is 15 years or less. The 15-year cutoff is somewhat arbitrary. To provide some context, this is roughly what remaining life expectancy was at age 65 in most low mortality countries around the beginning of the 1970s.

We call the chronological age at which remaining life expectancy falls to 15 years, the *prospective old-age threshold*. Now in our two-dimensional world, there are two threshold ages at which people first become categorized as being old. There is the conventional old-age threshold at age 65 (or perhaps 60) and the prospective one. The prospective old-age threshold varies across time, space, and population subgroups. The prospective old-age threshold tells us how old people need to be to be considered old, where the criterion for being categorized as old is having a remaining life expectancy of 15 years or less. For example, applying the prospective old-age threshold to Brazil, we would categorize people there as being old beginning at age 59.8 in 1950–1955, at age 68.8 in 2010–2015, and, using United Nations forecasts (United Nations 2017b), at age 77.4 in 2095–2100.

The three most commonly used measures of population aging are the *proportion of the population categorized as old (PO)*, the *old-age dependency ratio (OADR)*, and the *median age (MA)* of the population. These are measures that could be clearly perceived wearing eyeglasses where only one dimension is visible. When we enter the two-dimensional world, each of those measures has a prospective counterpart. There is a *prospective proportion* of the *population* who are categorized as being *old (PPO)*, which uses the prospective old-age threshold, the *prospective old-age dependency ratio (POADR)*, which also uses that threshold, and a *prospective median age (PMA)*, which uses prospective ages.

In Chapter 4, we address a practical question: Does it matter whether prospective or conventional measures are used to assess population aging? The answer is that the use of prospective measures dramatically changes our view of population aging. For example, in Brazil, the median age of the population (both sexes combined) was 19.0 years in 1953 and 30.2 years in 2013, an increase of over 11 years. During that same period, the prospective median age did not increase, but fell from 38.8 years in 1953 to 37.2 years in 2013. In Brazil, as elsewhere, our understanding of population aging in the past and its likely future path depends on which glasses we are wearing.

In Chapter 5, we show that prospective age is a special case of a more general concept that we call *α-age*. α-ages are ages based on various characteristics of people. Remaining life expectancy is one of these characteristics. When α-ages are based on remaining life expectancy, we obtain prospective ages. When α-ages are based on chronological age, they are just chronological ages. But α-ages can be computed based on many characteristics, such as hand-grip strength, walking speed, self-rated health, 5-year survival rate, and many others. Once different characteristics of people are translated into α-ages, they can all be compared and analyzed within a consistent framework, because they are expressed in the same units.

With our multidimensional glasses on, in Chapter 6, we explore the life cycle stage called "old age." When people, regardless of time, place, and their other characteristics, were categorized as being old at age 65, that age defined the beginning of the stage of old age. In that case, as life expectancy increased, the stage of old age lengthened. With our new vision, we categorize people as old based not on their chronological age but rather on their remaining life expectancy. Therefore, we have a different definition of the stage of old age. We present the features of the periods of old age defined using age 65 as the old-age threshold and using the prospective old-age threshold. We focus on two features, the proportion of adult years lived in old age, which we call the *life course ratio*, and health at the onset of old age, as measured by the 5-year survival rate.

Let's consider how long Italians live in old age. If we assume that old age begins at age 65, and that its onset will remain at that age throughout the century, we see (using United Nations forecasts) that in 2015–2020, 31 percent of all adult years lived by Italians (both sexes combined) would be in old age. However, the reward that the Italians will have from maintaining their good diets, living the good life, and continuing not to be bothered too much by their politicians is that, in 2095–2100, 39 percent of all their adult years would be lived in old age. We would feel sorry for the Italians, having to live such a large proportion of their adult years in the stage of old age, if we thought that age 65 was the right old-age threshold to use, but we do not. When we use the prospective old-age threshold, where old age begins at ages where remaining life expectancy is 15 years, we see something different. In 2015–2020, 20 percent of the adult life years of Italians would be spent in the stage of old age, and in 2095–2100 that percentage is 19 percent, virtually the same as in 2015–2020. The percentage of Italians' adulthood spent in the state of old age will be about the same for the entire century. Italians, you may continue what you are doing without fear that it will result in a much longer old age. In Chapter 6, we deliver the same message to people in many countries.

When we think of old age as being defined by the characteristics of people, not just their chronological ages, the onset of old age as a life cycle stage becomes something interesting to investigate. We show in Chapter 3 that the prospective old-age threshold increases over time as life expectancy increases. In Chapter 6, we show that 5-year survival rates at the prospective old-age threshold are forecast to fall very slowly in low mortality countries over the current century. To the extent that 5-year survival rates are related to health, then, the health of people just entering the stage of old age would be slowly improving over time.

In Chapter 7, we investigate healthy life expectancies at the prospective old-age threshold using detailed survey data on aspects of health including physical and mental activity limitations and self-assessed health. We find that the percentage of the remaining years of life in old age spent being healthy has been nearly constant or very slowly increasing. This is consistent with what we see in Chapter 6 using life table data. Health in the state of old age did not generally decrease in the early part of this century in the European countries where we can measure it, even though old age has been starting at older and older ages. What we see with respect to health is based on very limited data. Data for different time periods and countries may show a different picture and certainly the past is not necessarily a reliable predictor of the future. Nevertheless, the data that we have do not suggest that the stage of old age has been becoming a less healthy one over time.

Ever since Ballod's formulation in 1913, population aging has been conceptualized as changes in population age structures, the numbers of people at each age. With our new glasses, we can also see population aging from an additional perspective, one that is not dependent on age structures. This new view uses comparisons across countries, time, or both in age patterns of relevant variables. To experience this new way of seeing population aging, in Chapter 8 we travel to the Russian Federation and the United States where we look at trajectories of health across genders and ages. The trajectories we use are derived from a new kind of measure called *age differences*, differences between α-ages and chronological ages. Age differences provide information about how fast people in a population have aged relative to those in a reference population. Age differences are particularly useful in studying subgroups of populations. Using them, we explore the differences in patterns of aging in different places, including between people in Utah and Nevada, and between people in Moscow city and Moscow Oblast.

In Chapter 9, we use the concept of *age difference trajectories* and apply it to the study of gender differences in survival at older ages. For each gender, we compare patterns of survival to those observed in the country with the highest survival rates at the same time. Sometimes women are farther behind the best, sometimes men are. In terms of their relative position, we see that, in some countries, women had become more disadvantaged in terms of their survival over time.

As we walked around with our new glasses, we had many surprises. One of the greatest surprises was the discovery of the extent to which increases in life expectancy cause population aging. Using the three conventional measures, we show in Chapter 10 that there was faster population aging when there was an increase in life expectancy than when there was none. Using the prospective measures, to our surprise, we saw something completely different, that there was less aging when there was an increase in life expectancy than when there was none. In other words, breakthroughs that substantially slow the aging process would result in less population aging, even though they would increase the proportions of populations over 65 years old.

If increases in life expectancy slow population aging, is it possible that those increases would one day bring population aging to a halt? Might there one day be a future where populations are beyond aging even as life expectancy at older ages continued to increase? We would certainly not see this happening if we had one-dimensional vision, but we might see this when more dimensions are visible. We investigate this question in Chapter 11. Our approach is to compute conventional and prospective measures of population aging using United Nations population forecasts. What we found was there is no need for amazing breakthroughs to bring about the end of population aging. When we use our multidimensional glasses, we see that the end of aging is forecast to occur in many countries during this century and that in some, like China, population aging will be over in the next few decades.

Our new glasses also provide a new perspective on an important public policy question related to aging: How should the public pension age be determined? In Chapter 12, we define an intergenerationally equitable public pension age and show how it changes as life expectancy increases. Changes in pension ages are often justified by financial exigencies. If pension ages and pension amounts are thought to be appropriate, then countries have many ways of paying for them besides increasing pension ages and lowering pension payouts. We believe that a more appropriate way of thinking about pensions is to view them through the prism of intergenerational equity.

We define the intergenerationally equitable pension in a highly simplified model of a pension system based on Sweden's notional defined contribution plan. In the context of our simple model, we show that the calculation of the intergenerationally equitable pension age involves one of the characteristics derived from life tables that we discuss in Chapters 5 and 6, the life course ratio, the ratio of person-years lived from a given age onward to all adult person-years lived. We present the simple mathematics of determining intergenerationally equitable pension ages for a range of countries and use United Nations forecasts to show how they increase over time. The pace of the increase in the intergenerationally equitable pension age is similar to changes already legislated in a number of countries. Pension systems could contribute to intragenerational equity as well as intergenerational equity and in the appendix to the chapter, we show how this could be done again using the life course ratio.

There are significant differences between how we see population aging, when we wear eyeglasses that allow us to see in only one dimension or replace them with glasses that allow us to see in many dimensions. In the past, the only data that most statistical agencies produced were age structure measures that solely took chronological age into account. But now things are different. On the United Nations' website *Profiles of Ageing 2017* (United Nations 2017f), there are two old-age dependency ratios: the conventional one and the prospective one. It is highly unlikely that future discussions on population aging will take the form, "on the one hand, conventional measures show a certain amount of aging, but on the other hand, prospective measures show that the extent of aging will be very different." It is said that US President Harry Truman was once so annoyed with the economic advice in that vein that he told his chief of staff to bring him only one-handed economists in the future. So, in the spirit of President Truman, in Chapter 13, we explore the obvious question: Which old-age dependency ratio would a one-handed demographer recommend?

In our view, the study of aging is not fundamentally about how old people are. It is about people's capabilities and their disabilities. These things are not fixed according to chronological age. As life expectancy increases, the capabilities and disabilities of people at various ages change (Vaupel 2010). As life expectancy increases, the cognitive functioning of older people, at specific ages, tends to improve. Now, in many countries as life expectancy increases, national pension ages are also rising (OECD 2011). Changes in the age-specific characteristics of older people are observed everywhere from record-breaking performances in track and field events, to 70+ year-old rock stars performing to sell-out crowds, to the increasing labor force participation rates of 65+ year-olds in OECD countries. These changes are observable everywhere—except when people wear the old pair of glasses.

Here Are Your New Glasses

In this book, we present a new approach to conceptualizing and measuring population aging. A new approach is necessary because the old approach of ignoring all characteristics of people except their chrono-logical age is so obviously wrong. We need only look at the histories of increasing life expectancies to see this. So, if you are wearing the old, one-dimensional glasses, please take them off. We are happy to offer you a new pair of glasses and invite you to join us in traveling through the rich multidimensional demographic environment of population aging. We trust that you will be delighted at all the new and beautiful things that you will be able to see.

1

A Brief History of Measures
of Population Aging

At the heart of the study of population aging is the distinction between people and populations. Human populations are, of course, composed of people. People have life cycles and are born totally dependent. With good luck and appropriate care, people grow and mature. At some time, people enter a phase of declining physical and cognitive capacities, grow old, and eventually die. Populations, though, are not people. Over time, if people remain alive, they grow older, but populations can grow older or younger. People age, but populations do not have to. People rarely live more than 100 years, while many populations have survived for centuries. Populations are groups of people defined by a set of common attributes. A population could be women in Estonia in 2015 who had a college education. It could be men in Bangladesh in 1950 who lived in rural areas. What we see when we look at populations depends on the glasses that we are wearing.

We begin our journey together in Germany. This is where the conventional glasses through which population aging has been viewed and measured were first developed around a century ago. They were designed in a demographic and computing environment very different from what we experience today. In this chapter, we tell the history of one of the oldest of measures of population aging, the *total dependency ratio (TDR)*, and one of the most recent, the *economic support ratio*

(ESR). This history is limited by our language abilities and is focused primarily on the literature in English and secondarily in German. While we have tried to capture the highlights of the history, we have made no attempt at completeness.

Kārlis Balodis and the Total Dependency Ratio

The father of the oldest measure of population aging still in widespread use was the Latvian economic demographer Kārlis Balodis, although most of his books and articles were written in German under the name of Carl Ballod. The following history of Balodis draws heavily on "Der Zukunftsstaat: Carl Ballod's Vision of a Leisure-Oriented Socialism" (Balabkins 1978). Balodis attended the University of Tartu in what is now Estonia (then Russia). He received a Bachelor of Divinity degree in 1888, but, in addition to religion, Balodis also studied geography and statistics. For a while, Balodis went back and forth between academic and religious pursuits. In 1893–1895, he worked as a Lutheran minister in the city of Zlatoust, then part of the Ufa Governorate of the Russian Empire. Zlatoust, a city of around 20,000 people with a Lutheran minority, was a center of iron, steel, and weapons production (Wikipedia, n.d.e). His congregation was largely a group of German and Latvian workers in a rifle factory. Since Ufa was largely Christian Orthodox and Muslim (Wikipedia, n.d.d), it would have been unlikely that a Latvian- and German-speaking Lutheran minister would have lived there. Balodis's experiences in Zlatoust led him to give up the ministry and become a Marxist.

While in Zlatoust, Balodis collected demographic information, which later became the basis of a book coauthored with Dr. Ludvig von Besser entitled *Smertnostj, vozrastnoi sostav i dolgovechnostj pravaslavnogo norodonaseleniya oboego pola v Posssii za 1851–1890*, which translates to *Mortality, Age Composition, and Longevity of the Orthodox Population of Both Sexes in Russia, 1851–1890* (*Memoires de L'Academie Imperiale* 1897). With the success of that book, which won a prize from St. Petersburg's academy of sciences, Balodis embarked on a successful and productive academic career.

The central theme in Balodis's work was data-driven, rational planning. He, likely, would have felt very much at home in today's world of big data analyses. Among his many books, he wrote *Grundriss der Statistik, enthaltend Bevölkerungs-, Wirtschafts-, Finanz- und Handels-Statistik* (Statistical Outlines, including Demographic, Economic, Financial, and Commercial Statistics) (Ballod 1913). The book is a compendium of statistics on demography, the economy, finance, and commerce. There, we find on pages 30 and 31 the first version, to our knowledge, of what is now called the TDR.

Balodis (Ballod 1913) analyzed data from Austria, France, Germany, Italy, and the United States in 1900 or 1901. He divided their populations into five age groups, children (0–14), youths (15–19), prime age workers (20–59), adults with reduced work capacity (60–69), and the aged (70 and over). This age decomposition was used to produce a ratio of those who needed support to those who were in a position to provide the support. He called his ratios "coefficients of burden" (Belastungskoeffizienten in German). The people categorized as burdens were those 0–14 years of age and 70 years old or older. The people who were in the position to support them were those who were 20–59 years old. People 15–19 and 60–69 were assumed to be able to support themselves. To our knowledge, Balodis was the first to classify people into his five age groups, in order to approximate their need for or ability to provide support.

Balodis did not discuss why he chose 70 as the threshold at which he assumed elders became dependent. However, in 1889, Germany adopted the world's first national old age pension system. When Balodis wrote *Grundriss* in 1913, 70 was still the national pension age in Germany, so perhaps this was one motivating factor.

Balodis's coefficient of burden is a hybrid of two pure kinds of measures. One pure measure categorizes people as dependent and not dependent and expresses the ratio of dependents to nondependents. This form survives as today's TDR. Another pure form quantifies the extent of people's consumption and production. If people produce as much as they consume, they can be considered to be just supporting themselves. This is how Balodis treated people 15–19 years old and 60–69 years old. A version of this survives in today's ESR. The two, nevertheless, do not fit together well. If people aged 60–69 just support themselves, then shouldn't a person aged 59 produce only a bit more than is required to support himself? Shouldn't a person aged 70 produce just a bit less? But in the Balodis coefficient of burden, a person aged 59 is counted as being as productive as a person of 39 and a person of age 70 is counted as being as dependent as a person of age 90. The hybrid nature of Balodis's ratio is perhaps its most distinguishing feature and we will trace its appearance until it finally disappears in the 1940s. The entire presentation of the coefficients of burden took up only around 2 pages in a 348-page book. It was easy to overlook. Further, the book was not published at the best time to garner a wide readership. World War I broke out the year following publication, and Balodis himself was busy with other matters. He devised the system of rationing used in Germany during the war. Perhaps partially due to these factors, and possibly because of his Marxism, Balodis is not credited, in the English or the German demographic literatures, with producing the first TDR. His contribution is, however, recognized in the Russian-language literature.

The Total Dependency Ratio in the English Language

Balodis did not use his ratio to discuss the potential challenges of population aging. Concern about population aging emerged some years later. An early articulation of the challenge caused by population aging can be found in the work of two demographers, Warren Thompson and Pascal Whelpton. In 1930, they wrote an article entitled "A Nation of Elders in the Making" in which they foresaw how the age structure of the United States would be changing.

They wrote,

> We have been hearing a great deal of late regarding the attitude of industry and business in general toward men past forty. It appears that many firms have an absolute deadline at forty and will not consider hiring any one either in the factory or the office who is past that age. We shall not go into the whys and wherefores of this attitude, nor shall we inquire whether it is just and reasonable. We shall content ourselves here with pointing out that there will be a large and steady increase of persons over forty in our population during the next several decades. This fact is as certain as that the sun will rise tomorrow. We must, therefore, squarely face the problem of how these older people, whom the efficiency experts are now turning out, are

to be provided for so that they can maintain their self-respect and will not constitute a crushing burden upon the productive energies of younger people. (Thompson and Whelpton 1930, 393)

To clarify, by "turning out," Thompson and Whelpton mean that the efficiency experts are having people above the age of 40 fired from their jobs.

The same sort of analysis articulated by Thompson and Whelpton in 1930 has been repeated numerous times since. It has three parts. First, the number of older people is growing. For Thompson and Whelpton, the older people were those past the age of 40. Nowadays, it might be more like 60. Second, these older people would need to be supported by others and third, if no way could be found to keep older workers economically productive or less demanding, they would "constitute a crushing burden upon the productive energies of younger people." Nowadays, this burden is different from what it was in 1930. It is often discussed in terms of pension and healthcare costs, but nevertheless it is striking that the three-part structure of the argument is the same today as it was in 1930.

The three-part argument about aging that is so familiar today was followed in 1932 with its quantification. In 1932, Whelpton wrote,

The effect of the increasing proportion of elders on the problem of dependency is one that hinges in large measure on the extent to which persons can continue at productive work after they pass the best working ages. The large gain in the proportion of the population in the older age groups is at the expense of the younger age groups, as has been indicated, the 20–49 age period changing but little. There will be less children to be looked after and supported, but more older people, and because of smaller families there will be fewer brothers and sisters to share in caring for their aged parents. If persons 15–19 and 50–69 can be classed as only self-supporting and those under 15 and 70 or over as dependents who must be supported by producers 20–49, the ratio of dependents to producers is found to have declined from 869 per thousand in 1900 to 744 per thousand in 1930; and under the assumptions previously noted as to future population growth, the ratio of dependents to producers 20–49 will be 641 per thousand in 1950 and 684 per thousand in 1975. (Whelpton 1932, 99–100)

It is striking that this passage recounts almost exactly Balodis's hybrid formulation. Balodis treated people 0–14 as fully dependent, as does Whelpton in this passage. Balodis treated people 60 to 69 as being able to support themselves and Whelpton changed this to those 50 to 69. Correspondingly, the people who support others are 20–49 in the Whelpton version and 20–59 in Balodis's analysis. It is possible that the similarity of the two measures was coincidental, but it seems more likely to us that it wasn't. Whelpton had a strong interest in the German demographic literature (Whelpton 1935).

The passage from Whelpton in 1932 described a measure of population aging that, at that time, did not have a name in English, but it soon would. Within a decade, Whelpton's measure, or minor variations of it, would be called the "dependency ratio" (Cole and Lund 1941). Nevertheless, Whelpton's version of the Balodis ratio is not what we know today as the TDR.

Today's Total Dependency Ratio and Old-Age Dependency Ratio

Today's form of the TDR was likely a simplification of Balodis's formulation as brought into the English literature by Whelpton. It was clearly articulated in 1944 in a volume entitled *The Future Population of Europe and the Soviet Union: Population Projections, 1940–1970* (Notestein et al. 1944) that was written for the League of Nations.

The TDR was the ratio of those classified as dependents to those classified as potential supporters. The dependents were those 0–14 years old and those 65 years old or older. The people who could support them were those ranging from 15 to 64 years old. The hybrid feature, people considered as just able to support themselves, of the Balodis-type measures was gone. The TDR in Notestein et al. (1944) is still one of the measures of population aging that the United Nations uses today. A formal mathematical definition of the TDR and other measures of population aging appear in the mathematical appendix to this chapter.

Also appearing in Notestein et al.'s publication was a graph of the *old-age dependency ratio (OADR)*. Today, the OADR is commonly defined as the ratio of people 65 years old and older to those in the "working ages," usually 20 to 64 or 15 to 64.

Notestein et al. (1944) garnered a great deal of attention for its clear exposition and analysis of comparable demographic projections for a variety of countries, which were headed for quite different demographic challenges after World War II. This successful collaboration of demographers with the League of Nations was an important element in the establishment of the Population Division within the Department of Economic and Social Affairs of the United Nations in 1946. The first director of that division was Notestein himself and the TDR and the OADR as defined in Notestein et al. (1944) remain commonly used measures of aging produced by the United Nations and many other statistical agencies today.

The establishment of the United Nations Population Division was a watershed in the estimation, forecasting, and analysis of the population age structures of nations. Its challenge was to produce the same sort of analysis that appeared in Notestein et al. (1944) for all of its member states. Some countries had good demographic data, but most did not. To quantify age structure change required the estimation of age structures and their histories for many countries. This was an unprecedented challenge, somewhat akin to reconstructing a zoo full of extinct animals, each from a different set of bones. The United Nations Population Division overcame this challenge and there now exists population age structure estimates for virtually all countries of the world from 1950 to today at 5-year intervals.

Notestein et al. (1944) wrote about the populations of European countries, including the Soviet Union, and based their findings on population projections over the period of 1940 to 1970. In defining the TDR, they reminded their readers:

> Any age limits set for the productive and dependent groups are bound to be inadequate for the heterogeneous area and the thirty-year period under consideration. Nevertheless, uniformity of treatment requires some arbitrary limits to be set. (Notestein et al. 1944, 153)

The United Nations (United Nations 2017c) now publishes 5 different TDRs with fixed chronological ages. The youngest in the working-age population could be 15, 20, or 25. The oldest in the working-age population could be 64 or 69. Nevertheless, the warning about arbitrary age limits is still relevant today.

Ernst Günther, the Inventor of Today's Economic Support Ratio

Balodis's version of the TDR quantified differences in age structures across countries in a new way based on existing data. In retrospect, his quantification seems natural and Balodis himself spent little time discussing it. In contrast, the ESR was invented in 1931 by Ernst Günther in a 52-page paper entitled "Der Geburtenrückgang als Ursache der Arbeitslosigkeit? Untersuchung einiger Zusammenhänge zwischen Wirtschaft und Bevölkerungsbewegung," which translates to "The Decline in Births as a Cause of Unemployment? An Investigation into the Relationship between Economic and Demographic Changes" (Günther 1931). It presented an entirely new measure of population aging and, for its time, was a brilliant analysis of it. We do not know whether Günther ever read *Grundriss* or whether he paid much attention to Balodis's coefficient of burden, but we do know that Günther knew, at least, about some of Balodis's writing. Indeed, in 1919, he wrote an entire pamphlet severely criticizing one of Balodis's later books (Balabkins 1978).

In Balodis's coefficient of burden, people are divided into three types according to their age, either they are net burdens, net producers, or neither because their burden and production balance out. Günther's view was much more nuanced. Instead of dividing people into groups according to age, he understood that people are often both producers and consumers and that productive capacity and consumption demands varied with age. There are two innovations here. First, people were no longer conceptualized as burdens. Yes, at some ages people consume more than they produce, but the language of "burden" provides an interpretation of this difference that Günther avoided. The second innovation is the recognition that it was important to consider the entire age pattern of production and consumption, not just whether one was larger than the other.

Today's ESR stems from Cutler et al. (1990). Although they were unaware of it, Cutler et al. (1990) reinvented Günther's ratio, which at the time was over half a century old. The United Nations' version of the ESR is based on data created in the National Transfer Accounts project (NTA, n.d.a). This amazing project has merged standard economic accounts with life cycle generational accounting. Among many other variables, the NTA project has produced age profiles of labor income and consumption. The ESR uses these data and is computed as the ratio of the number of standardized producers to the number of standardized consumers. The number of standardized producers at each age is the per capita labor income of people of that age divided by the average per capita labor income of people aged 30–49. The number of standardized consumers at each age is the per capita consumption of people of that age also divided by the average per capita labor income of people aged 30–49. The ESR has the desirable feature that it is not based on fixed ages. Production and consumption profiles differ across countries and years.

The most obvious difference between Günther's ESR and the current one is that the labor and consumption schedules in Günther's are gender-specific. Günther had an advantage here because his ratio did not need to be based on detailed observations. Plausible approximations were all that were needed for his analysis, just as in the case of Cutler et al. (1990). Recently, gender-specific information has been added to NTA data for some countries and more will follow (Agenta, n.d.; NTA, n.d.b). In the future, ESRs will include gender-specific flows and look a bit more like their 1931 predecessor.

There are minor differences between Günther's ESR and the current one. In the current ESR per capita labor earnings are computed relative to those of people 30–49 years old. In Günther's ratio productive capacity is computed relative to that of 25–40-year-old men. Women at each age are assumed to be two-thirds as productive as men. In the current ESR, consumption is computed relative to the income of 30–49-year-olds. In Günther's it was computed relative to the consumption of 20–50-year-old men. Women in that age group are assumed to consume 80 percent as much as men. At younger and older ages, the consumption of women is assumed to be closer to that of men. None of these differences in standardization change the underlying conceptualization of aging expressed in the ratios of standardized production units to standardized consumption units.

Günther's ESR was an entirely new conceptualization of the relationship between age structure change and economic performance. Detailed observations on the age patterns of production and consumption

did not exist in 1931, so Günther had to rely on plausible approximations. Günther showed that his ratio rose in Germany from 1910 to
1930. To our knowledge, this was the first time that the changes over
time in an indicator of aging were computed and analyzed. Günther's
interpretation of what he saw, however, is surprising. Currently, increases in the ESR are often associated with faster economic growth
and fewer challenges from an aging population (Mason et al. 2017).
Günther argued, to the contrary, that the increase in his support ratio
was one of the causes of the increase in unemployment in Germany.

When Günther wrote his article, Germany had experienced a decade of massive unemployment. Günther argued that, in an environment of weak demand, having more people in prime working ages does
not increase output; it just increases unemployment. Günther showed
that the implications of changes in the support ratio depended on economic circumstances. To our knowledge, Günther's paper provided the
most comprehensive analysis of the relationships between age structure change and economic performance that had been published up to
that time.

Thompson and Whelpton (1933) cite Günther's paper and show the
implications of it using historical data for the United States from 1870 to
1930 and their medium forecasts for 1950 and 1980. The ESR in Thompson
and Whelpton (1933) had one advantage over Günther's. Thompson and
Whelpton (1933) were able to use data on the age profile of earnings in
the United States that had been collected earlier (Sydenstricker and
King 1921).

Like Günther, Thompson and Whelpton are clear about the age profile weights that are used to create the numbers of standardized producers and consumers. They wrote,

> Many faults can be found with any such set of weights. All that is
> claimed for these is than they are fairly reasonable in light of such
> facts as are available and help to measure the economic effects of the
> age changes during the period covered. (Thompson and Whelpton
> 1933, 169)

In 1933, the United States was also experiencing massive unemployment, and this was reflected in their discussion of their ESR.

The general bearing on employment of this relative increase of productive units would seem to be in the direction of making it more difficult to find work unless consumption is so changed as to take up the slack. There should be no difficulty in accomplishing the latter because an improvement in standards of living has come to be regarded as normal. However, it will be noted that the above conclusion is based on the assumption that people at the several ages will actually be in a position to use their productive power. (Thompson and Whelpton 1933, 169–170)

It is interesting to compare the visions of Balodis and Günther. According to Balodis, increases in the number of older people cause an increasing burden on those who support them. According to Günther, increases in the number of people who could support the elderly, could cause an increase in their unemployment when there are not enough jobs for them. It follows that an increase in the number of elderly people could result in a decrease in unemployment because of its effects on the demand for labor. In our view, Balodis and Günther could both be correct under some circumstances and this suggests caution in interpreting measures of aging out of context.

Conclusion

Most measures of aging in use today are related to the pioneering work of Balodis and Günther. By 1933, versions of their measures of aging had already appeared in English. Balodis's coefficient of burden seems to have evolved into today's TDR and OADR, while Günther's version of the ESR was forgotten and independently reinvented.

If people familiar with the literature on population aging in the 1930s were shown much of what is written about population aging today, they would have no difficulty understanding it. The measures are basically the same today as they were then. But the world is different now. Life expectancy has increased substantially, the data available to analyze population aging has expanded dramatically, and the computing power to do analyses has exploded. It is time to view population aging from a twenty-first-century perspective.

Mathematical Appendix

Balodis's coefficient of burden (BCB) can be written as

$$BCB_{i,t} = \frac{\sum\limits_{a=0}^{110+} v_a \cdot N_{a,i,t}}{\sum\limits_{a=0}^{110+} w_a \cdot N_{a,i,t}}.$$

$BCB_{i,t}$ is the Balodis coefficient of burden in place or group i in year t, v_a is a vector of age-specific coefficients that are 1 for people in the dependent age groups 0–14 years old and 70 years old or older and 0 for everyone else; w_a is a vector of age-specific coefficients that are 0 for people 0–19 and 60 years and older and 1 for everyone else; $N_{a,i,t}$ is the number of people at age a in place or group i; t is the year; and the highest age group considered is people 110 years old and older.

The formula for computing the *total dependency ratio (TDR)* has the same form as the BCB with small differences in the v_a and the w_a coefficients.

$$TDR_{i,t} = \frac{\sum\limits_{a=0}^{110+} v_a \cdot N_{a,i,t}}{\sum\limits_{a=0}^{110+} w_a \cdot N_{a,i,t}},$$

where $TDR_{i,t}$ is the total dependency ratio in place or group i in year t; v_a is a vector of age-specific coefficients that are 1 for people in the "dependent age groups" 0–19 years old and 65 years old or older and 0 for people in the "working ages" 20–64; w_a is a vector of age-specific coefficients that are 0 for people in the dependent ages and 1 for those in the working ages; $N_{a,i,t}$ is the number of people at age a in place or group i; t is the year; and the highest age group considered is people 110 years old and older.

For us, a key feature of both the BCB and the TDR is that neither the v_a nor the w_a coefficients have a subscript related to time or place.

Günther's economic support ratio (GESR) can be expressed as

$$GESR_{i,t,s} = \frac{\sum\limits_{a=0}^{75+} \sum\limits_{g=1}^{2} v_{a,g,s} \cdot N_{a,g,i,t}}{\sum\limits_{a=0}^{75+} \sum\limits_{g=1}^{2} w_{a,g,s} \cdot N_{a,g,i,t}},$$

where $GESR_{i,t,s}$ is the value of the Günther's economic support ratio in country i in year t; $v_{a,g,s}$ is the productive potential of someone of age a and gender g relative to that of men in the age group of 25–40 (using the baseline productivity schedule s); $w_{a,g,s}$ is the consumption demand of someone of age a and gender g relative to that of men 20–50 (using the baseline consumption schedule s); and $N_{a,g,i,t}$ is the number of people of age a and gender g in country i in year t.

The coefficients $v_{a,g,s}$ and $w_{a,g,s}$ are age- and gender-specific and reflect standard patterns of production and consumption that do not change over time.

The *economic support ratio (ESR)* uses age profiles of labor income and consumption produced in the National Transfer Accounts project (NTA, n.d.a). In form, it is a simplification of the GESR:

$$ESR_{i,t,s} = \frac{\sum\limits_{a=0}^{99+} v_{a,i,s} \cdot N_{a,i,t}}{\sum\limits_{a=0}^{99+} w_{a,i,s} \cdot N_{a,i,t}},$$

where $ESR_{i,t,s}$ is the economic support ratio for country i in year t using weights from standard year s, and $N_{a,i,t}$ is the number of people at age a, in country i in year t. The United Nations (2015) describes $v_{a,i,s}$ as the standardized number of workers at age a, in country i in standard year s, and $w_{a,i,s}$ as the standardized number of consumers at age a, in country i in the standard year s.

The standardized number of workers at age a, in country i in year s is the per capita labor income of people of age a in country i in the base year s divided by the arithmetic mean per capita labor income of people 30–49. The standardized number of workers, then, does not depend on a count of people who are working. The $v_{a,i,s}$ coefficients are more accurately described as standardized levels of per capita labor income in the base year. The standardized number of consumers at age a, in country i in year s, is the per capita consumption of people of age a in country i in the base year s divided by the arithmetic mean of per capita labor income of people 30–49.

2

Prospective Ages

The Human Life Cycle: Looking Backward and Looking Forward Simultaneously

We have moved from Germany to Rome and are enjoying la dolce vita in the Forum Holitorium. We are here because this was once the site of a temple to the Roman god Janus. Among other things, Janus was the Roman god of doorways and beginnings, so there is no better place to put on our new glasses and begin to experience the multidimensional view of population aging. Janus is depicted as having two heads, one looking forward and one looking backward. Our challenge in this chapter is to apply what Janus sees to the study of population aging. It is to expand the concept of age into a two-dimensional notion, making it more relevant in a world of changing life expectancy.

When we wrote our first article on aging (Sanderson and Scherbov 2005), we were building on an article by Lee and Goldstein (2003) that addressed what Janus might see as life expectancy increased. They called their hypothetical framework "proportional life cycle rescaling" and wrote,

> Proportional rescaling of the life cycle, in which every life cycle stage and boundary simply expands in proportion to increased life expectancy, provides a convenient benchmark. Under proportional rescaling, if longevity doubles, then so would childhood, the length of

work and retirement, the span of childbearing, and all other stages of the life cycle. Proportional rescaling of the life cycle would appear to be neutral in some sense, so that life, society, and economy could continue as before, except that there would be proportionately more time spent in every stage. However, we will find that while this is (or could be) true for some aspects of life, other aspects would vary with the square or some other power of longevity. (Lee and Goldstein 2003, 183)

In 2005, we reasoned that in a world in which life cycle stages become rescaled with changes in life expectancy we needed an additional measure of age, one that considered changes in life expectancy. The traditional measure of age is chronological age. This is a person's backward-looking age; it is how many birthdays a person has already celebrated. This measure tells only part of the story. The lifespan ahead of the person is ignored. Like Janus, who is looking forward and backward at the same time, people can look back at the life that they have lived and forward to what lies ahead of them. So, in 2005, to complement the traditional backward-looking age, we developed a forward-looking one. We call this *prospective age* and it is calculated based on *remaining life expectancy*. It took us a while to become comfortable with seeing population aging through the lens of prospective age. Nowadays, it is hard for us to remember how we used to see things and we apply the adjective *prospective* to any measure of aging that is adjusted based on remaining life expectancy.

The importance of people's backward-looking and forward-looking ages depends on where they are in their life cycles. For 5-year-olds, for example, it does not matter much whether they have 60 or 70 years ahead of them. For older people, the amount of remaining time becomes more important. Conventional measures of population aging use only characteristics that are fixed according to backward-looking age. It is as though one of the heads of Janus was blindfolded so he could no longer look forward. When we remove the blindfold, a new dimension of age becomes visible, one that is changing over time and is different from place to place.

Life Expectancy Schedules

The relationships between remaining life expectancies and chronological ages are published by several organizations, including the United Nations, Eurostat, the United States Census Bureau, and the Human Mortality Database. In particular, the United Nations has produced estimates of remaining life expectancies from age 0 to 100 and over for virtually every country in the world from 1950–1955 to 2010–2015 and forecasts to 2095–2100. Clearly visible in that dataset is that, over the last half century, life expectancy at 65 in high-income countries has increased at a rate of about one and half years per decade. The rate has increased even faster in many other countries.

The relationships between remaining life expectancy and chronological age are often published as columns in life tables. The tables organize mortality data to produce life expectancies and other important mortality indicators. We call the relationships between remaining life expectancies and chronological ages *life expectancy schedules*. Figure 2.1 shows the life expectancy schedules for 40–80-year-old women in France for the years 1950–1955, 2015–2020, and 2095–2100 using the United Nations' data. For each period, the life expectancy schedules are downward sloping, indicating that remaining life expectancy decreases with chronological age. Over time, however, the curves shift upward, indicating that people at the same chronological age have a higher remaining life expectancy if they were born later.

If we look at the life expectancy schedule for French women in 1950–1955, we see that 60-year-olds had a remaining life expectancy of 18.35 years and 70-year-olds had a remaining life expectancy of 11.20 years. In 2015–2020, the life expectancy of 60-year-old French women would be 27.86 years, almost a decade longer than their counterparts in 1950–1955 and 70-year-old women would have a remaining life expectancy of 19.14 years about 8 years longer than women of the same age in 1950–1955. Using the United Nations' forecasts of French survival rates in 2095–2100, we see that 60-year-old French women would have a remaining life expectancy of 36.04 years, about twice the remaining life expectancy that women of the same age had in 1950–1955. In 2095–2100, 70-year-old French women have a forecasted

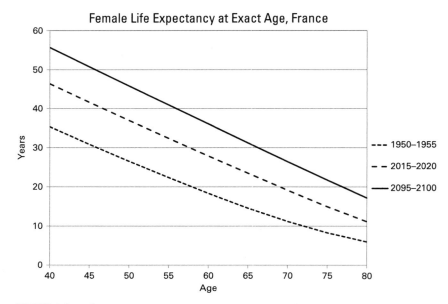

FIGURE 2.1: Life expectancy in France, women 40–80, 1950–1955, 2015–2020, 2095–2100.

Data source: United Nations (2017e).

remaining life expectancy of 26.40 years, which implies that around half of them would survive to their 96th birthdays (70 plus 26.4).

Life expectancy schedules are also different for different countries at a point in time. We show this in Figure 2.2, where we compare the life expectancy schedules in India, France, and Brazil for 40- to 80-year-old women in 2015–2020. The French curve is the highest, indicating that at any specific chronological age, French women have a higher remaining life expectancy than Brazilian or Indian women. For example, at age 60, French women had a remaining life expectancy of 27.86 years, Brazilian women 23.65 years, and Indian women 18.86 years.

Calculating Prospective Ages from Two Perspectives

Prospective ages can be computed from two different perspectives. The two different perspectives are a bit like viewing a mountain that rises

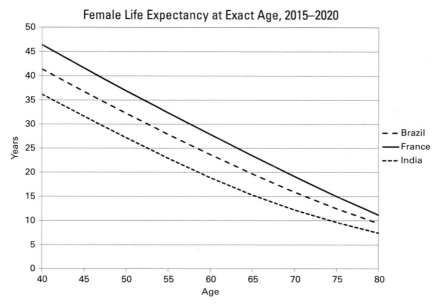

FIGURE 2.2: Life expectancy in India, France, and Brazil, women 40–80, 2015–2020.

Data source: United Nations (2017e).

above a beautiful valley. We can look at the majesty of the mountain tops from the valley and we can look at the mountain tops from high on the mountain itself. The mountain tops remain the same but exactly what we see depends on where we are standing.

We describe the two perspectives using Table 2.3, which is based on the observed remaining life expectancies of Japanese women reported in the Human Mortality Database (HMD) (University of California, Berkeley, and Max Planck Institute for Demographic Research 2017).

In 1972, 50-year-old Japanese women had a remaining life expectancy of 29 years. In 2014, the latest year for which HMD data for Japan are available at this writing, 50-year-old Japanese women had a remaining life expectancy of 38 years. Fifty-year-old Japanese women in 1972 and 2014 had the same chronological age, but they had different remaining life expectancies. This is similar to what we saw in

Figure 2.1 for French women. For each chronological age in that figure, remaining life expectancy increased with the passage of time.

In Figure 2.3, we see the life cycles of Japanese women in two dimensions; we see how many years they have already lived and how many years they are expected to live in the future. Using the old set of glasses, however, we cannot see the differences in remaining life expectancy. It is as if, in Panel A of Figure 2.3, Janus's forward-looking head was blindfolded. He could see that 50-year-old Japanese women in 1972 and 2014 had lived the same number of years, but he could not see that they had different remaining life expectancies. With his forward-facing head blindfolded, Janus could only see that all 50-year-olds look the same regardless of when they lived, where they lived, or anything else about them.

In the study of population aging, an important characteristic of people is their remaining life expectancy. When the blindfold is removed from Janus's forward-looking head, he can see both of the panels of Figure 2.3. He can read Figure 2.3 in two ways. First, he can see that 50-year-old Japanese women in 1972 had lived the same number of years as 50-year-old Japanese women in 2014, and, in addition, he can see that 60-year-old women in 2014 had the same remaining life expectancy as 50-year-old women in 1972. When age functionally depends on people's average remaining life expectancy, then Janus can see that 60-year-old women in Japan in 2014 are functionally as old as 50-year-olds in 1972 because they have the same remaining life expectancy. If we compare Japanese women in 2014 with those in 1972, we can say that the 60-year-old Japanese women in 2014 had a prospective age of 50 because those 60-year-old women had the same remaining life expectancy as 50-year-old women in 1972.

The second way that Janus could read Figure 2.3 is based on a fixed value of remaining life expectancy. For example, in Figure 2.3, if a remaining life expectancy of 29 years was a fixed characteristic of interest, we could say that 50-year-old Japanese women in 1972 and 60-year-old Japanese women in 2014 had equal prospective ages because they all had the same remaining life expectancy of 29 years. Sometimes, we will need to distinguish prospective ages computed from the different perspectives. In those cases, we will call constant characteristic ages based on a fixed value of remaining life expectancy *prospective constant char-*

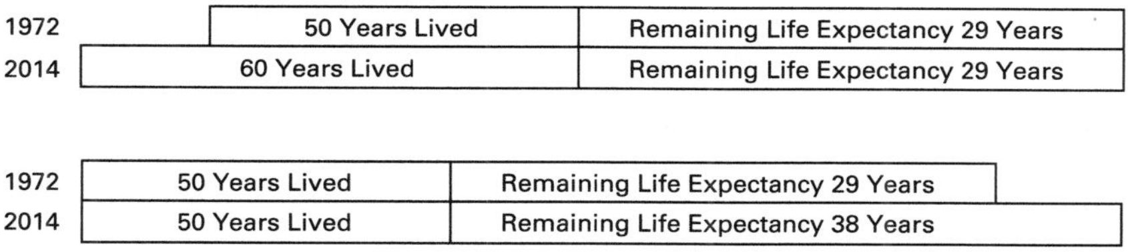

1972	50 Years Lived	Remaining Life Expectancy 29 Years
2014	60 Years Lived	Remaining Life Expectancy 29 Years

1972	50 Years Lived	Remaining Life Expectancy 29 Years
2014	50 Years Lived	Remaining Life Expectancy 38 Years

FIGURE 2.3: Schematic representation of the computation of a prospective age, Japanese women 1972 and 2014.

Data source: University of California, Berkeley, and Max Planck Institute for Demographic Research (2017).

acteristic ages. Prospective ages are always comparative. Exactly how the comparison is made is largely a matter of expositional convenience.

Computing a Prospective Age from a Chronological Age

Now, let us look at Figure 2.3 again, this time step by step. We do this in Table 2.1. In the first step, we chose to compute the prospective age of 60-year-old Japanese women in 2014 using 1972 as the year of comparison. So, we put age 60 in the left-most column and to its right we put the remaining life expectancy of 60-year-old Japanese women in 2014. That remaining life expectancy is 29 years. The final step is finding the age at which Japanese women in 1972 have a remaining life expectancy of 29 years. It is at age 50. The prospective age of 60-year-old Japanese women in 2014 is 50, using the Japanese population of 1972 as a standard of comparison, so we write 50 in the right-most column.

Figure 2.3 and Table 2.1 were constructed to show an example where 60 was the new 50 (50 and 60 are nice round numbers and it seemed that their use made it clearer that we were presenting an example, rather than if we were to have shown a case where 62 was the new 47). We started with Japanese women in 2014, the latest year for which Japanese data were available (at this writing). In 2014, Japanese women had the highest life expectancy at birth among women in all countries of the world. Because of their comparatively high life expectancies, the Japanese often serve as a standard of comparison in this book. The year 1972 was chosen because that was the year when remaining life expectancy at age 50 was the same as at age 60 in 2014.

Table 2.1 Example of the calculation of the prospective age of 60-year-old Japanese women in 2014 using Japanese women in 1972 as a standard of comparison

Chronological age—Japanese women 2014	Remaining life expectancy—Japanese women 2014	Remaining life expectancy—Japanese women 1972	Prospective age—Japanese women 1972
60	29	29	50

Data source: University of California, Berkeley, and Max Planck Institute for Demographic Research (2017).

At first, Table 2.1 might seem a bit disconcerting, because there is an age in the left-most column and another age in the right-most. It is almost as if we were seeing double. This is not a mistake. It is our intent to open this second parallel world to exploration. For the moment, seeing people for the first time as having two ages, a backward-looking chronological age and a forward-looking prospective one, might leave some readers a bit queasy but probably not those who have had a course in economics.

The concept of measuring economic magnitudes in two dimensions is part of the standard undergraduate economics curriculum and is so frequently incorporated into economic discussions that it is barely noticed. Almost all measures of economic output come in two forms, one unadjusted for inflation and another adjusted for inflation. For example, the gross domestic product of Canada in 2015 was 1.561 trillion Canadian dollars when measured in current prices. When measured in the prices of 2007 it was 1.376 trillion (Statistics Canada 2016). Economists would have no problem with gross domestic product being either 1.561 trillion Canadian dollars or 1.376 trillion Canadian dollars depending on the prices used.

The computation of prospective ages and the computation of economic magnitudes adjusted for inflation are similar. To adjust an economic magnitude for inflation, a baseline set of prices is chosen. To adjust demographic magnitudes for changes in life expectancies, we do a similar thing using a baseline life table. Prospective age is just chronological age indexed to take changes in life expectancy into account.

There is no going back to the old, one-dimensional demographic world now. It would be like asking economists to go back to a world in which they could not see any inflation-adjusted figures.

Looking at Figure 2.3 and Table 2.1, the new two-dimensional world may begin to appear more familiar. After all, phrases such as "60 is the new 50" are in common usage. They are informal examples of prospective ages, indicating that 60-year-olds today behave like 50-year-olds in some previous time. In essence, the schedule of the relationship between age and behavior at the previous time serves as a standard schedule. We observe the behavior of 60-year-olds today and find that equivalent behavior was exhibited by 50-year-olds in the past. Fifty is the prospective age of today's 60-year-olds using the past schedule of the relationship between behavior and age as a standard. This is what we showed in Figure 2.3 and Table 2.1. Phrases like "60 is the new 50" were in common use before the concept of prospective age was invented. People have already been walking in the two-dimensional demographic environment. Prospective age just provides a GPS to help us navigate in it.

In the process of providing people with a prospective age, we get a bonus, which is the difference between their prospective age and their chronological age. The difference is the advantage or disadvantage in terms of remaining life expectancy that people in one population have compared to people in the other. For example, in Figure 2.3 and Table 2.1, Japanese women at age 60 in 2014 had the same remaining life expectancy as 50-year-old Japanese women in 1972 (29 years), so the difference between the prospective and chronological age is 10 years.

Prospective Ages of 65-Year-Old Women and Men

In Figure 2.3 and Table 2.1, we were computing a single prospective age. We did this to help readers feel more comfortable with their new glasses. Now, let us do some exploring. In Table 2.2, we show the prospective ages of 65-year-olds in 30 countries. For consistency, when we compute prospective ages for many countries, it is helpful to use a single standard for each gender. In Table 2.2, we use the Japanese life tables for men and women in 2010–2015 as standards. Japanese women had the highest remaining life expectancy at age 65 in 2010–2015 in the United Nations' life table database (23.91 years), so all prospective ages for women have to be above age 65. Japanese men at age 65 in 2010–2015 had high life expectancies (18.98 years), but there were a few countries in the world where life expectancies for men were a bit higher.

In Table 2.2, we see that in Germany the prospective age of 65-year-old German women in 2010–2015 was 68.54. This means that,

Table 2.2   Prospective ages of 65-year-olds in 2010–2015 in different
             countries using Japanese life tables in 2010–2015 as standards

Country	Female	Male	Gender difference
Australia	67.02	64.56	2.46
Austria	68.04	66.32	1.73
Brazil	70.10	68.51	1.59
Costa Rica	68.56	65.87	2.69
France	66.09	64.93	1.16
Germany	68.54	66.83	1.71
Iceland	68.22	65.00	3.22
India	75.53	71.95	3.58
Indonesia	76.54	74.36	2.18
Israel	68.12	64.99	3.14
Italy	67.15	65.55	1.60
Kazakhstan	74.97	75.17	−0.20
Kenya	75.09	71.36	3.73
Malaysia	73.45	70.25	3.20
Mexico	69.82	66.34	3.48
Netherlands	68.22	66.42	1.80
Nigeria	81.06	76.79	4.27
Pakistan	76.31	71.54	4.77
Poland	69.90	69.69	0.21
Republic of Korea	67.40	66.98	0.42
Russian Federation	72.83	73.24	−0.41
Singapore	67.32	65.49	1.83
South Africa	75.14	75.89	−0.76
Swaziland	77.12	74.81	2.31
Thailand	70.52	68.31	2.21
Turkey	71.30	70.54	0.77
United Arab Emirates	73.15	68.99	4.15
United States of America	68.82	66.23	2.58
Vietnam	68.74	69.09	−0.36

Data sources: United Nations (2017e); authors' calculations.
Note: Remaining life expectancy for 65-year-old Japanese women in 2010–2015 was 23.91 years and for men was 18.98 years.

given the United Nations' life tables, Japanese women would get to live 3.54 years (68.54 minus 65) after age 65 before their life expectancy fell to the level of 65-year-old German women. 65-year-old German men in 2010–2015 had a prospective age of 66.83. Japanese men in 2010–2015 would have the same remaining life expectancy as 65-year-old German men in that period when they reached the age of 66.83. The higher prospective age is above chronological age, the lower is remaining life expectancy compared to the Japanese. Countries in Table 2.2 where women's remaining life expectancies at age 65 are relatively low, and, therefore, their prospective ages are relatively high, include Brazil, Egypt, India, Indonesia, Kazakhstan, Kenya, Malaysia, Nigeria, Pakistan, the Russian Federation, South Africa, Swaziland, Thailand, Turkey, and the United Arab Emirates. The countries where women do well relative to the Japanese are Australia, Austria, France, Italy, the Republic of Korea, and Singapore. Countries that have high prospective ages for women, and, therefore, relatively low remaining life expectancies, tend also to have them for men. Three countries stand out as having especially high prospective ages for women compared with those for men—Nigeria, Pakistan, and the United Arab Emirates. Using prospective ages, we can see that women in those countries are particularly disadvantaged relative to their male compatriots.

Prospective Ages Based on Constant Remaining Life Expectancies

In Figure 2.3 and Table 2.1, we showed how to start with a chronological age and compute the corresponding prospective age. In Table 2.3, we again use data for Japanese women in the Human Mortality Database. We start with a remaining life expectancy of 29 years, which was the same one that we used in Figure 2.3 and Table 2.1. Table 2.3 shows the ages at which Japanese women had a remaining life expectancy of 29 years. In 1972 that remaining life expectancy was reached at age 50. In 1994, it was reached at age 56 and, in 2014, it was reached at age 60.

Table 2.4 provides some examples of prospective ages based on a constant remaining life expectancy of 15 years. The lowest prospective age in the table is for Nigeria, where 58.4-year-old people had a remaining life expectancy of 15 years. The next lowest are two other

Table 2.3   Ages based on a constant remaining life expectancy of
29 years, Japanese women, 1972, 1994, and 2014

Remaining life expectancy	1972	1994	2014
29 years	Age 50	Age 56	Age 60

Data source: University of California, Berkeley, and Max Planck Institute for
Demographic Research (2017).

African countries, South Africa and Madagascar, but both have prospective ages more than 3 years higher than Nigeria's. Japan has the
highest age at a remaining life expectancy of 15 years. People there
had to be almost 74 before they had a remaining life expectancy of
15 years. People with the same prospective constant characteristic age
have the same remaining life expectancy. Therefore, in terms of remaining life expectancy, we can see that 58.4-year-old Nigerians in
2018 were forecasted to be as old as 73.9-year-old Japanese. We will discuss an important application of prospective constant characteristic
age in Chapter 3.

Table 2.4   Chronological age at a remaining life expectancy of 15 years,
both sexes combined, selected countries, 2018

Country	Age at remaining life expectancy of 15 years
Brazil	69.6
China	66.6
Egypt	63.7
Germany	71.3
India	64.5
Japan	73.9
Madagascar	63.0
Netherlands	71.4
Nigeria	58.4
Russian Federation	65.5
South Africa	62.6
United States	71.5

Data source: United Nations (2017e).
Note: The figures are based on the forecasted 2015–2020 life tables.

Janus and Our New Vision of Population Aging

In this chapter, we have begun to explore what we can see with two-dimensional vision. For good reasons, we will probably never get to the day when people will answer the question "How old are you?" with another question: "Are you asking about my chronological or prospective age?" The question "How old are you?" means "How many years have you lived?" But for the study of population aging, how many years people have lived is only one of their characteristics. People are complex beings, and in the study of population aging, we need to know more about them. With our two-dimensional vision, like Janus, we can now see entire lifetimes, with the past quantified as people's chronological ages and their futures quantified as their prospective ages.

Even if one accepted the argument that, in the study of population, it is useful to supplement chronological age with a forward-looking analog, the question would remain about whether prospective age was the best supplement. After all, it is simpler just to think about people in the two dimensions of years lived and average years left to live, chronological age and remaining life expectancy.

The use of prospective age has two main advantages over this simple approach. First, prospective age is inherently comparative. When we say someone has a prospective age of 60 using Japanese women of 2000 as a standard, we are saying that this person has the same remaining life expectancy as 60-year-old Japanese women in 2000. The second reason is prospective age is a special case of the multidimensional view of population aging that we will present later in the book. People have many characteristics that are relevant to the study of population aging, such as their activity limitations and self-rated health. The same approach that we presented here, translating remaining life expectancy into prospective ages, works more generally by converting characteristics expressed in quite different units into a common metric: age.

When people say things like "60 is the new 50," they are providing examples of both advantages. The phrase "60 is the new 50" compares people of age 60 in one place or time with 50-year-olds in another. If Janus were to look forward from age 60 in one population, he would see people behaving like 50-year-olds in the other. "60 is the new 50" compares people in two populations, not just in terms of their remaining life expectancy, but in terms of many of their behaviors and characteristics.

But we are getting ahead of the story here. Readers will have to wait until Chapter 5 to experience the full multidimensional view of aging available with the new glasses.

Mathematical Appendix

In this appendix, we provide a graphical explanation of the computation of *prospective ages* from chronological ages and the computation of *prospective constant characteristic ages*.

The Computation of Prospective Ages, Given a Chronological Age

Figure 2.A1 has three life expectancy schedules. One, labeled *St*, shows the *standard schedule.* The other two schedules, labeled I_1 and I_2, indicate the index schedules, schedules for populations 1 and 2, respectively. The computation of the prospective ages starts by specifying a chronological age. In Figure 2.A1 that chronological age is denoted as

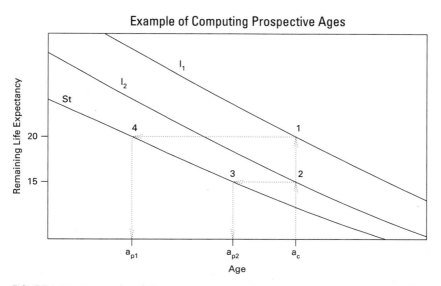

FIGURE 2.A1: Example of the computation of prospective age starting with a chronological age.

a_c and is the same for each of the two index relationships. What we want to do is to find the prospective ages of people with chronological age a_c in each of the two populations.

People of age a_c in population 1 have a *remaining life expectancy* at point *1*. To find the age in the standard schedule with the same remaining life expectancy, we move horizontally from point *1* to point *4*. The age in the standard schedule with this remaining life expectancy is a_{p1}. This is the prospective age of people at age a_c in population 1 using the *standard population* as a basis of comparison. Repeating the same procedure for population 2, we would begin again at a_c. Life expectancy at a_c in population 2 is at the point labeled 2. We find the age in the standard schedule with the same remaining life expectancy by moving horizontally to point *3*.

In Figure 2.A1, the standard population has relatively low remaining life expectancies. Population 2 has higher remaining life expectancies and population 1 has even higher ones. The prospective age of someone in population 2, a_{p2}, is lower than a_c, indicating that people in the standard population reach the same remaining life expectancy as those at

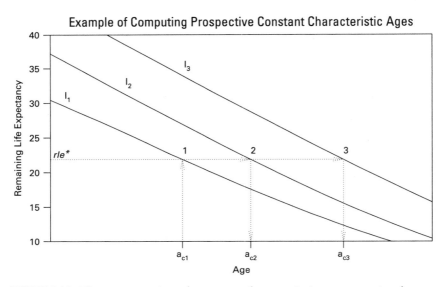

FIGURE 2.A2: The computation of constant characteristic ages, starting from a specific level of the characteristic.

age a_c, in population 2 at a younger age. People in the standard population age faster than those in population 2 because it takes them fewer years for their remaining life expectancy to fall to the same level. Population 1 has higher life expectancies than population 2 and correspondingly the prospective age a_{p1} is lower than a_{p2}.

The Computation of Prospective Constant Characteristic Ages

In Figure 2.A2, we show how prospective constant characteristic ages, the chronological ages of people with a fixed remaining life expectancy, are calculated. We plot the life expectancy schedules for three populations. Figure 2.A2 is different from Figure 2.A1 in that no distinction is made between standard and index populations. In Figure 2.A2, we start with a fixed remaining life expectancy labeled rle^*. The chronological ages of people in the three populations with that remaining life expectancy are found by drawing horizontal lines to where they intersect the life expectancy schedules. This happens at points labeled [1], [2], and [3], and the corresponding chronological ages are labeled a_{c1}, a_{c2}, and a_{c3}. Those are three prospective constant characteristic ages associated with the level of remaining life expectancy rle^*.

3

How Old Do You Need to Be to Be Old?

WITH OUR NEW glasses on, we travel westward from the Forum Holitorium in Rome to Arnhem in the Netherlands, where we are enjoying a cup of *warme Chocolademelk* (hot chocolate). At this writing, a district court in Arnhem has just ruled on a case brought by Emile Ratelband, a 69-year-old motivational speaker. Mr. Ratelband had sued the Dutch government to change his age officially to 49. He argued that physically and mentally he is more like a 49-year-old and that his chronological age leaves him vulnerable to all sorts of discrimination and makes it less likely that he would find an appropriate partner on internet dating websites. Mr. Ratelband also argued that older people are now functionally different from what older people were like in the past and that this difference should be reflected in their official ages (Domonoske 2018; Brueck 2018).

The district court ruled against Mr. Ratelband saying that laws stipulate people's rights and privileges in terms of their chronological ages and, therefore, changes in those ages would render those laws inoperative. Mr. Ratelband is certainly correct in arguing that the functioning of older people has changed, and the court is certainly correct in that the timing of rights and privileges associated with old age cannot be specified differently for each individual. When age is viewed as having a single dimension, this conflict is difficult to resolve. With our new glasses, there is no conflict. People have both a chronological age and a *prospective age*. The rights and privileges associated with old age can be defined in terms of prospective age and, therefore, reflect the changing functioning of people. This does not entirely respond to Mr. Ratelband's suit. Prospective age is a population-based concept, not an individual one. Nevertheless, perhaps Mr. Ratelband would get more internet dates if he included his prospective age in his personal profile.

Mr. Ratelband certainly does not consider himself to be old, but he is old enough to receive a pension from the Dutch government and other rights and privileges associated with his chronological age. For legal and administrative purposes, it is convenient, even necessary, to have some age at which people begin to be classified as old. However, this threshold age is not appropriately applied to individuals. People do not suddenly become old from one day to the next. But old-age thresholds do exist and form an important element in many public policies and business practices. Mr. Ratelband's suit raises the question of how old-age thresholds should be defined in an environment where people are living longer and healthier lives.

This chapter is devoted to answering that question. We proceed in five steps. First, we look at a few illustrative stories about old age at the level of the individual. The second step is to investigate aging at the population level by studying patterns of life expectancy change. The third step is to report on what some demographers, economists, and historians have said on the topic of when people could be categorized as being old. Fourth, we will look at how the insights from the first three steps are reflected in conventional measures of population aging. Finally, we will look at the beginning of old age through our new glasses.

Stories of Old Age at the Individual Level

On September 23, 2015, Hidekichi Miyazaki competed at the Kyoto Masters Competition one day after his 105th birthday (Himmer 2015). He was a relative newcomer to athletic completions. He only took up running in his early 90s. Immediately after he completed the 100-meter sprint, he said (in translation), "I'm not happy with the time. I started shedding tears during the race because I was going so slowly. Perhaps I'm getting old!" (*Japan Times Online* 2015). On that day Miyazaki ran the 100-meter sprint in 42.22 seconds. His time was disappointing because he had run the sprint 6 seconds faster in training. But even his training time would not have been a record in the 100-meter sprint in the 105–109-year-old group. On June 28, 2015, Stanislaw Kowalski ran the 100 meters in 34.50 seconds in Torun, Poland. At that time, Kowalski was 77 days older than the disappointed Miyazaki. He also took up running only in his 90s. On the same day as Kowalski's record-breaking run, he also set records in the shot put and discus. This was not surprising. He was the only person over 105 years old to have competed in those events (Groom 2015).

The organization that keeps track of these sorts of records is called the World Masters Athletics (World Association of Masters Athletes, n.d.). Its record book shows that stories like those of Miyazaki and Kowalski are not unique. New age groups for both men and women continue to be added to the record book. In April 2017, Man Kaur's performances required that the World Masters Athletics record book add a new category for 100–104-year-old women. At this writing, Man Kaur holds the records for the 100-meter sprint, the 200-meter sprint, shot put, and javelin in that age group. She began her involvement in athletics at age 93. Her trainer at the time she set those records was her 79-year-old son (Grund and Lewis 2017).

Then there is Sister Madonna Buder, known as the Iron Nun. Her nickname derives from her accomplishments in Ironman athletic competitions. In 2016, at age 86, she became the oldest woman to complete an Ironman triathlon (Triathlon Inspires, n.d.; Wikipedia, n.d.b). That triathlon required a 2.4-mile swim, followed by a 112-mile bicycle ride, and then a 26.2-mile run without a break. Completing the triathlon would be quite a feat even for people half her age.

Even without glasses, we see older people running, swimming, and biking faster. Others, like the Rolling Stones, are entertaining people in sold-out concerts around the world. At this writing, all members of the Rolling Stones were over 70 years old.

Patterns of Life Expectancy Change at Age 65

Our understanding of how to set the boundary of old age at the population level depends on understanding the changes in life expectancy. The United Nations has produced an amazing dataset of life table estimates and forecasts for virtually every country in the world from

1950–1955 to 2095–2100. Using these life tables, we can observe life expectancies by age and gender as well as other variables of interest.

In Figure 3.1, we provide some of the numbers that we see in those life tables—*remaining life expectancies at age 65* for men in Chile, India, the Netherlands, and the Russian Federation from 1950–1955 to 2095–2100. We chose these countries because of the differences and changes in their patterns of life expectancy that they exhibit. Our focus here is not on any country or region but on a new way of viewing population aging in general.

In Figure 3.1, we can see that 65-year-old men in Chile, the Netherlands, and the Russian Federation had somewhat similar remaining life expectancies at age 65 in 1950–1955. Over time, the life expectancies of Chilean and Dutch men grew more rapidly than those of Indian and Russian men. Importantly, we see that the remaining life expectancy of 65-year-old Russian men fell from 1950–1955 to 2000–2005. The United Nations forecasts that by the end of the century the life expectancy of 65-year-old Russian men will be well below that of men in Chile and the Netherlands.

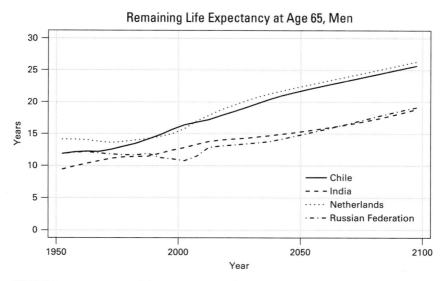

FIGURE 3.1: Remaining life expectancy of 65-year-old Chilean, Indian, Dutch, and Russian men.

Data source: United Nations (2017e).

The Onset of Old Age in the Academic Literature

Life expectancies have generally been rising for many decades, and this has been clearly visible in the United Nations life table database (United Nations 2017e) and the Human Mortality Database (University of California, Berkeley, and Max Planck Institute for Demographic Research, 2017). No special glasses are needed to see this trajectory. It is clearly visible that the experience of aging is not the same everywhere. In this section, we provide examples from the academic literature on how this is perceived.

Thane discussed aging from a historical perspective:

> Contemporary discourse about the global aging of populations, especially in relation to the costs of health and social care and the impact upon social and economic conditions, tends to be alarmist in tone, partly because it often assumes the experiences of aging and later life to be unchanging historical constants. It is often assumed that the experience of the present can be extrapolated into the future. For example, the proportion of physically or mentally impaired 80-year-olds in the year 2000 will be the same in 2050 and, hence, the absolute numbers will be, alarmingly, much greater. This is to underestimate change in the experience of aging over time, to fail to recognize that the physical and mental condition of one cohort of 80-year-olds may be very different from another because their life experiences have been different. To take one example, an 85-year-old living in Western Europe today will have been born in the middle of World War I in the vastly poorer economic circumstances of most European populations in the early twentieth century. He or, more probably, she will have experienced the economic depression during the nineteen twenties and thirties, which in many countries was prolonged and severe. She would have lived through the trauma of World War II. She would have been in her forties before the prosperity of the later twentieth century became part of her everyday experience. On the other hand, a woman born in 1945 and reaching the age of 80 in 2025 will have had very different and generally less traumatic experiences, though not all of them are yet known. Among other things, she will have benefited from the advances in medicine from the mid-twentieth century. The future is hard to predict, but examining the past and change over time can help us to guard against serious pitfalls of prediction. (Thane 2001, 1)

Neugarten (1996) noted that the changing characteristics of the elderly interacted with public policies. She wrote,

> I noted that despite the fact that age is becoming less useful or less relevant in addressing adult competencies and needs, we have witnessed a proliferation of policy decisions and benefit programs in which target groups are defined on the basis of age, a trend that is particular evident with regard to older people. (10)
>
> I persist, nevertheless, in believing that all of us, young and old, would be well ahead if policymakers would focus not on age, but on more relevant dimensions of human competencies and needs. (11)

It is too bad that Neugarten did not survive to witness Ratelband's suit. Our guess is that she was the type of person who would have enjoyed testifying in it.

Lowsky et al. (2014) took a more quantitative approach. They wrote,

> For a surprisingly large segment of the older population, chronological age is not a relevant marker for understanding, measuring, or experiencing healthy aging. Using the 2003 Medical Expenditure Panel Survey and the 2004 Health and Retirement Study to examine the proportion of Americans exhibiting five markers of health and the variation in health-related quality of life across each of eight age groups, we find that a significant proportion of older Americans is healthy within every age group beginning at age 51, including among those aged 85+. For example, 48% of those aged 51–54 and 28% of those aged 85+ have excellent or very good self-reported health status; similarly, 89% of those aged 51–54 and 56% of those aged 85+ report no health-based limitations in work or housework. (640)

Over 4 decades ago and well before the passages above were written, Ryder (1975), one of the giants of twentieth-century demography, had already provided a quantitative old-age threshold that was not a universal constant. He wrote,

> Once past youth, we tend to associate age with various bad things that happen to each of us individually, despite our recognition that aging is better than its alternative. As a society, we applaud the lengthening of the average lifetime but are dismayed by the aggregate consequences, in large part because our institutional structure is ill-designed to accommodate those in the upper reaches of the life

span. One dimension of the problem deserves re-examination. We measure age in terms of the number of years elapsed since birth. This seems to be a useful and meaningful index of the stages of development from birth to maturity.

Beyond maturity, however, such an index becomes progressively less useful as a clue to other important characteristics. To the extent that our concern with age is what it signifies about the degree of deterioration and dependence, it would seem sensible to consider the measurement of age not in terms of years elapsed since birth but rather in terms of the number of years remaining until death. . . . We propose that some arbitrary length of time, such as 10 years, be selected and that we determine at what age the expectation of life is 10 years, that age to be considered the point of entry into old age. . . . What this does is substitute for the fixed age 65 a lower limit for "old age" which depends on the level of survival. It is proposed as a valid reflection of vital reality-a measure of the health implications, at ages prior to death, of raising the mean age at death. (Ryder 1975, 15–16)

Using the terminology in this book, in 1975 Ryder recommended the use of an old-age threshold based on a fixed prospective age instead of a fixed chronological age. We call old-age thresholds based on a fixed remaining life expectancy or equivalently a fixed prospective age *prospective old-age thresholds.*

When Ryder wrote the passage above in 1975, demographers were primarily interested in problems associated with rapid population growth rather than population aging, and, to our knowledge, even Ryder himself never published another word about his suggested old-age threshold, nor did any of the authors just cited.

The first applications of Ryder's old-age threshold to observed data was in 1984 by Siegel and Davidson, appearing in one table in a report with more than a hundred other tables. In that report, Siegel and Davidson wrote,

The concept of years until death could serve as the basis for a new measure of individual aging. Specifically, the demarcation line for "old age" could be a variable line which recognizes the fact that, as life expectancy increases, old age starts at increasingly higher ages. Such a linkage of the definition of old age to changing longevity may be a basis for defining old age in programs where funding is affected by the length of life (e.g., Social Security benefits). Life expectancy of older persons has increased greatly (4 years) since the Social Security Act went into effect in 1938, and if the proportion of the population covered by Social Security must be kept at the same level, one device for achieving this is to shift the age at which full benefits are initially paid gradually upward to correspond to the changes in life expectancy. (Siegel and Davidson 1984, 14)

Siegel and Davidson computed dynamic old-age thresholds for the United States for 1920 to 1980 at 10-year intervals (Siegel and Davidson 1984, 18, table 2-10). In our terminology, their old-age thresholds were chronological ages associated with two levels of remaining life expectancy, 10 and 15 years. Siegel also applied Ryder's idea in Siegel (1993).

Ryder and Siegel approached the topic of computing an old-age threshold from a demographic perspective. Around the same time that Siegel and Davidson published their report, Fuchs, an economist, also joined the conversation about defining old age, apparently unaware of Ryder's earlier contribution. He wrote,

> The definition of old age—that is, the age of eligibility for retirement and Medicare benefits—is a critical variable in the development of viable programs for the elderly. . . . It is conventional to define the elderly with reference to the number of years since birth, but this is largely a concession to administrative convenience rather than the logical result of a closely reasoned argument. Individuals "age" at very different rates and, in theory at least, the elderly could be defined in terms of years until death, e.g., those men and women who will die within some specified time. . . . To be sure, it doesn't make much sense to define infants, children, and young adults as "elderly," even if they are close to death. But a count of persons aged 65 and over who will die within the next several years is informative because much of the interest in the elderly revolves around their need for medical care and other special services. (Fuchs 1984, 145)

Fuchs's definition of who is old is programmatic. Fuchs (1984) suggested three definitions of who is old: (1) everyone over 65, (2) everyone who is 65+ years old and within 5 years of death, and (3) everyone who is over 65 and not in the labor force. The second definition produces a number which changes as survival rates change. In contrast to Ryder

(1975) and Siegel and Davidson (1984), Fuchs did not suggest that the threshold of old age itself be made dynamic.

Over 3 decades later, Fuchs's colleague in the Department of Economics at Stanford University, John Shoven, ultimately defined an explicitly dynamic old-age threshold. Based only on Fuchs's 1984 paper, Shoven wrote,

> I argue that there are better alternatives to the standard measure of years-since-birth. In fact, I claim that public policy would be better if age were more appropriately specified in the law. A particularly simple alternative to years-since-birth would be a measure of age based on mortality risk. Groups whose mortality risk is high would be considered old, those with low mortality risk would be classified as young, and those with the same mortality risk would be considered to be the same age. Another closely related approach would be to measure age from the other end of life, at least in expected terms. That is, remaining life expectancy (RLE) would be the measure of age—those with a short RLE would be considered elderly and those with a long RLE would be considered young. One advantage of the RLE approach is that it is measured in years, units that are widely understood, unlike mortality risk, which is measured in the percentage chance of dying within a year. (Shoven 2010, 17)

In the passage above, Shoven suggested two possible old-age thresholds: one based on a fixed remaining life expectancy and another based on a fixed mortality risk. The first is the same as our prospective old-age threshold. We will address Shoven's second threshold in Chapter 5.

Fuchs and Shoven were primarily interested in the interaction of the concept of age and public policy. Historians, on the other hand, had a broader perspective on the issue. Bourdelais wrote,

> The comparison of the proportion of persons aged 60 and over at the end of the eighteenth century, the beginning of the twentieth and today hardly makes sense because "elderly" persons are currently so different in their destiny, life expectancy, position in the successive generations and state of health. Who would argue that the human reality designated by the category "old people of 60 and above" evolved very little between 1850 and 1930, and did not change radically in the past half century? Who would claim that studying the proportion of persons aged 60 and over since the eighteenth century

Table 3.1   Old-age thresholds for French men and women in selected years from 1825 to 1985

	1825	1860	1900	1910	1927	1937	1947	1957	1966	1975	1985
Men	59.6	60.2	59.2	59.3	60.6	60.6	63.7	63.5	64.0	65.1	67.4
Women	60.4	61.0	62.4	62.6	64.4	65.5	68.0	68.2	70.4	71.9	73.9

Source: Excerpted from Bourdelais (1998, 121, table 6.1).

could make the population's multicentury evolution intelligible? (Bourdelais 1998, 119)

Bourdelais computed a compound old-age threshold for France based on 5-year survival rates and remaining life expectancy. His old-age thresholds for years from 1825 to 1985 are shown in Table 3.1, and, to our knowledge, provide the longest, demographically consistent old-age thresholds ever published. According to his figures, the old-age threshold for men increased by 7.8 years from 1825 to 1985 and by 13.5 years for women. The figures in the table show that women and men entered the stage of old age at about the same chronological age in 1825, but by 1985, women entered that stage 6.5 years later than men.

The Old-Age Threshold Used in Most Measurements of Population Aging Today

It is clear that demographers, economists, and historians have long been pondering the timing of old age. Our next step is to see how their insights and analyses have been incorporated into the measures of population aging that are generally used today. We begin by looking at the history of the United Nations' old-age threshold.

According to the United Nations' *Vienna International Plan of Action on Aging,*

> Only in the past few decades has the attention of national societies and the world community been drawn to the social, economic, political and scientific questions raised by the phenomenon of aging on a massive scale. . . . In 1950, according to United Nations estimates, there were approximately 200 million persons 60 years of age and over throughout the world. (United Nations 1983)

Over 3 decades later, in the United Nations' *World Population Ageing 2015,*

> According to data from World Population Prospects: the 2015 Revision (United Nations, 2015), the number of older persons—those aged 60 years or over—has increased substantially in recent years in most countries and regions, and that growth is projected to accelerate in the coming decades. (United Nations 2015)

At the time of the *Vienna International Plan of Action on Aging* in 1983, using United Nations' life tables aggregated for the entire world, remaining life expectancy at age 60 (both sexes combined) was around 17.3 years. In 2015, it was around 20.4 years. The United Nations counted people as being old when they reached their 60th birthday. It did not matter what country they lived in or whether they were alive in 1950 or were expected to be alive in 2050. Life expectancy or any other characteristic of people simply did not matter. A chronological age 60 has been the United Nations' traditional old-age threshold for decades.

Old-age thresholds are, of course, concepts pertaining to populations, not to individuals. It's not that one's hair suddenly turns gray on one's 60th birthday. Imprecise as they are, old-age thresholds reflect something real about the human life cycle. People who are lucky enough to survive eventually do enter a life cycle phase that can be called "old age." Fixing the old-age threshold at a chronological age of 60 says that 60-year-old people in India in 1950, for example, should be treated as being functionally the same as 60-year-old people in Japan, for example, in 2050. This stands in contrast to the stories of how individuals age commonly reported in the news, in contrast to the evidence on increasing life expectancies and in contrast to the arguments made by demographers, economists, and historians about old age.

In the past, the most frequent fixed old-age thresholds have been age 60 and age 65. Age 65 was used in the dependency ratios in Notestein et al. (1944; see Chapter 1 for a history of dependency ratios and implied old-age thresholds) and is currently the most frequently used old-age threshold in those measures. The United Nations also uses age 60 as the old-age threshold when computing the proportions of populations who are counted as old. Bourdelais (1998) suggests that the use of 60 as the old-age threshold comes from a centuries old French and British demographic tradition. That tradition may well have stemmed from 60 being the age at which men were considered no longer fit for military duty. Thus, the two old-age thresholds used by the United Nations, age 60 and age 65, appear to have resulted from the adoption of two different preexisting demographic traditions.

The United Nations Population Division has been very creative in its demographic work. It often constructed population sizes, and age and gender distributions of populations, from fragmentary data. It made innovations in the probabilistic forecasting of populations. In 2017, the United Nations Population Division made history again by incorporating one of our measures of population aging, one based on our prospective old-age threshold.

The History of Our Approach to an Old-Age Threshold

Our approach to an old-age threshold evolved slowly. Our first paper devoted specifically to population aging was published in *Nature* in 2005, entitled "Average Remaining Lifetimes Can Increase as Human Populations Age" (Sanderson and Scherbov 2005). That was the first paper in which we used the concept of prospective age, although we called it there "standardized age." The paper's title refers to our finding that it is possible for *prospective median ages (PMA)* of populations to decrease over time even as median ages increase. In other words, in a population with a longer life expectancy, it is possible for the median-aged person both to be older than the median-age person in the population with a shorter life expectancy and have a longer remaining life expectancy. As a visual representation, picture a rubber band with a mark in the middle. As the rubber band stretches (life expectancy increases), the mark simultaneously gets farther from the left end (birth) and simultaneously farther from the right end (death).

In 2005, we were not interested in the idea of an old-age threshold and were unaware of any of the academic work in the area. In retrospect, we did indirectly address the issue. We presented projections of *total dependency ratios* for Germany, Japan, and the United States.

First, those ratios assumed two transition ages: people below the age of 20 and 65 and over were categorized as dependents. We then adjusted those ages from 2000 onward proportionally, based on the United Nations forecasts of life expectancy at birth, and computed new old-age dependency ratios to the end of the century.

In Sanderson and Scherbov (2007), we addressed technical issues relating to *prospective age.* Toward the end of the 2007 paper, we introduced a new old-age dependency ratio that we called the *prospective old-age dependency ratio (POADR)* and presented forecasts again for Germany, Japan, and the United States. The onset of old age in our article was a constant characteristic age based on the remaining life expectancy at age 65 in the country in the year 2000. This was the first time that we computed a time-varying age based on a constant characteristic.

In February 2008, we published probabilistic population forecasts over the twenty-first century for the major regions of the world in the journal *Nature,* comparing conventional and prospective measures of population aging (Lutz, Sanderson, and Scherbov 2008). Among the measures that we presented were the median age and the prospective median age. In addition, we presented forecasts for the proportion of the population over 60 years old, the conventional proportion old, and the proportion of the population in age groups with remaining life expectancy 15 years or less, the *prospective proportion who are considered old (PPO).* Ever since, we have used the chronological age at which remaining life expectancy falls to 15 years as an old-age threshold.

Later in 2008, we published a less technical article for the Population Reference Bureau (Sanderson and Scherbov 2008). In the draft submitted to the Population Reference Bureau, we included a discussion of our old-age threshold. An astute reviewer noted that it was exactly what had been previously published in Ryder (1975) and repeated in Siegel and Davidson (1984) and Siegel (1993). By a rather circuitous path, in 2008, we had independently reinvented what Ryder, Siegel, and Davidson had suggested decades earlier. In our research on population aging, we had not set out to find a useful old-age threshold, but the logic of our work on prospective age eventually led us to one anyway.

Prospective Old-Age Thresholds

In Figures 3.2, 3.3, and 3.4, we graph our prospective old-age thresholds for three pairs of countries, Brazil and Chile, India and China, and Nigeria and South Africa. In 1950–1955, the prospective old-age threshold in Brazil was 59.8 and in Chile it was 61.4. Half a century later, the prospective old-age threshold had risen by 7.3 years and 8.2 years in Brazil and Chile, respectively. Using the United Nations' estimates and forecasts, we see that over the 100-year period 1950–1955 to 2050–2055, the onset of old age was postponed by 14.4 years in Brazil and 13.6 years in Chile. Over the period 2010–2015 to 2095–2100, the prospective old-age threshold increases by about 1 year per decade in both countries. In 1950–1955, the prospective old-age threshold was 53.5 in China and 54.2 in India. From 1950–1955 to 2000–2005, the prospective old-age threshold increased by 11.4 years in China and 8.1 years in India. In Nigeria and South Africa, the prospective old-age thresholds in 1950–1955 were close to those in China and India but, subsequently, they increased

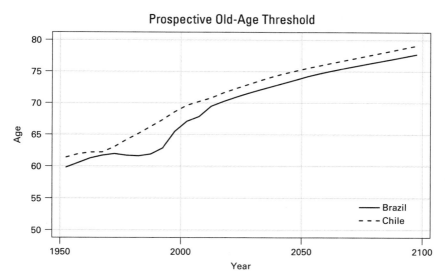

FIGURE 3.2A: Prospective old-age threshold, Brazil and Chile, 1950–1955 to 2095–2100, both sexes combined.

Data sources: United Nations (2017e); authors' calculations.

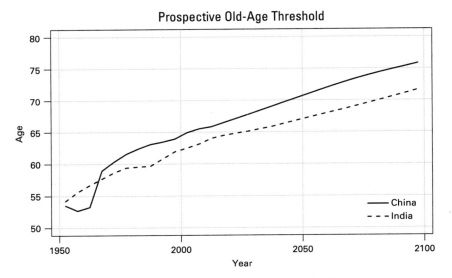

FIGURE 3.2B: Prospective old-age threshold, China and India, 1950–1955 to 2095–2100, both sexes combined.

Data sources: United Nations (2017e); authors' calculations.

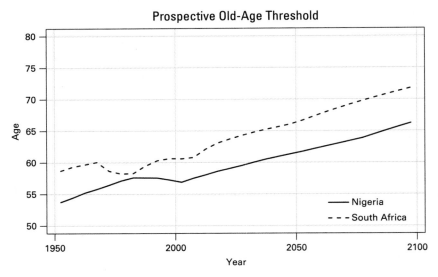

FIGURE 3.2C: Prospective old-age threshold, Nigeria and South Africa, 1950–1955 to 2095–2100, both sexes combined.

Data sources: United Nations (2017e); authors' calculations.

much more slowly. Strikingly using the United Nations forecasted life table for 2095–2100, the prospective old-age threshold in Nigeria would only be 66.2, which is about what it was in Chile in 1980–1985.

Wearing our old glasses, old-age thresholds looked like horizontal lines at age 60 or 65. There was no need to graph them for separate countries or even over time. The old-age threshold was fixed everywhere and forever at an unchanging chronological age. But this is not at all what we see in Figures 3.2a, 3.2b, and 3.2c. Prospective old-age thresholds differ from country to country and over time. Prospective old-age thresholds reflect the changing characteristics of people. The conventional old-age threshold does not.

Plausibility of the Prospective Old-Age Threshold

There are many possible ways to think about old-age thresholds. Inevitably, there will always be some arbitrariness in its definition. Therefore, it is useful to have some way to assess potential thresholds. Possible old-age thresholds can be evaluated using four criteria: ease of computation, plausibility, insensitivity of implications to plausible changes in assumptions, and usefulness.

First, setting the old-age threshold at the chronological age at which remaining life expectancy is 15 years is extremely simple when life tables are available. It is only necessary to read off the age associated with a remaining life expectancy of 15 years.

An old-age threshold should yield results that are plausible. We have two pieces of evidence here. According to a 2015 study of British adults by Cigna Insurance Services, people 50–64 reported that they thought that old age began at age 71 (Cigna 2015a, 2015b, 2015c). At the time of this writing, the last life table for the UK available from the Human Mortality Database was for 2013 (University of California, Berkeley, and Max Planck Institute for Demographic Research 2017). In 2013, remaining life expectancy at age 71 (both sexes combined) was 15.75. So, the prospective old-age threshold based on a remaining life expectancy of 15 years and the information on the onset of old age in the Cigna survey are consistent with one another.

Another piece of evidence, concerning on the plausibility of using a remaining life expectancy of 15 years to compute an old-age threshold, comes from a study by the Pew Research Center in the United States. In 2009, the center did a survey on attitudes toward aging (Taylor 2009). On average, 50–64-year-old respondents said that old age began at 72. In the 2009 United States life table from the Human Mortality Database, the remaining life expectancy of 72-year-old Americans (both sexes combined) was 14.22 years. This is again roughly consistent with our use of a 15-year remaining life expectancy.

The British and United States survey results show that the use of a remaining life expectancy of 15 years is, at minimum, not implausible. Had we instead chosen to use a remaining life expectancy of 20 years, the old-age threshold would have been 64.5 in both the United Kingdom (2013, both sexes combined) and in the United States (2015, both sexes combined) (University of California, Berkeley, and Max Planck Institute for Demographic Research 2017). Had we instead chosen to use a remaining life expectancy of 10 years, the old-age threshold would have been 78.3 years old in the United Kingdom (2013, both sexes combined) and 79.0 in the United States (2015, both sexes combined) (University of California, Berkeley, and Max Planck Institute for Demographic Research 2017). The old-age thresholds using either a remaining life expectancy of 10 years or 20 years seem less plausible to us and are less consistent with the survey results.

The third criterion for assessing old-age thresholds is whether some change, such as using a remaining life expectancy of 10 years instead of 15 matters. We have investigated this and found that none of our major findings are affected by the exact number we use for remaining life expectancy in the range between 10 and 20 years.

The fourth criterion is the usefulness of the old-age threshold. In the chapters that follow, we show that it is indeed useful and informative.

Conclusion

Old-age thresholds should take the changing characteristics of people into account. The only way to do this in a consistent way for a large number of countries and a long span of time is to use information derived from life tables. Given this limitation, the method that seemed most natural to us was to define the onset of old age based on remaining life expectancy. As a practical matter, any life table characteristic that we had used to define the onset of old age would give essentially the same results. The only way to get very different results is to be blind to the changing characteristics of people.

It is better to wear glasses that allow us to see realistic old-age thresholds than to be blind to them. But does seeing those old-age thresholds really improve our perception of population aging? To answer this question, we must travel around the demographic environment and see what things look like with our new glasses and without them.

4

How Different Are Measures of Population Aging Based on Chronological and Prospective Age?

IN CHAPTER 2, we provided readers with a new pair of glasses. With these, readers could see that people had both a chronological age and a *prospective age.* In Chapter 3, we focused on a particular prospective age, called the *prospective old-age threshold,* the age at which we suggest that people begin being categorized as old. In this chapter, we make use of our new glasses by taking a quick trip around the world to see what difference the new glasses make in our perception of population aging.

The study of population aging begins with the definition and quantification of a relevant magnitude. Every one of these measures of population aging is based on a set of assumptions. In particular, the conventional measures assume that all the pertinent characteristics of people do not change over time. In this book, we challenge this assumption. The three most widely used measures of population aging are the *proportion of the population categorized as being old (PO),* the *old-age dependency ratio (OADR),* and the *median age (MA).* In this chapter, we compare changes in those three measures with changes in analogous measures based on prospective age, the *prospective proportion who are considered old (PPO),* the *prospective old-age dependency ratio (POADR),* and the *prospective median age (PMA).* We also present a measure of aging that, to our knowledge, was never previously studied, the proportion of people 65 years old or older who are considered old.

Proportions of the Population Old

Do we see population aging any differently if we use the conventional measure of the proportion old or the prospective one? To answer that question, we compare the two measures for Brazil, Japan, and South Africa in Figures 4.1a, b, and c. The countries show three different patterns of aging. The conventional PO is the fraction of the population at or above the conventional old-age threshold (assumed to be age 65) and the PPO is the fraction of the population at or above the prospective old-age threshold (the age at which remaining life expectancy is 15 years).

In Figure 4.1a, we see that in Brazil, both the PO and the PPO were low and relatively stable for the second half of the twentieth century. Around the beginning of the twenty-first century, they were both around 0.05. After that, they both began to increase, but the rise is

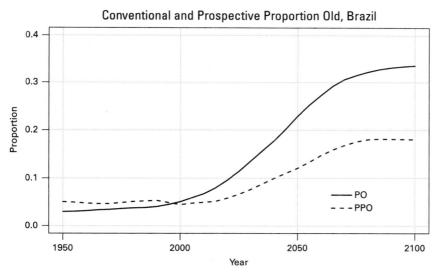

FIGURE 4.1A: Conventional and prospective proportions old, Brazil. Life tables for 5-year intervals are assumed to be close approximations to life tables at the midpoints of the 5-year intervals. Populations are interpolated to the midpoints of 5-year intervals. The proportion old (PO) and the prospective proportion old (PPO) are the same in the year when remaining life expectancy at age 65 is 15 years.

Data sources: United Nations (2017c); authors' calculations.

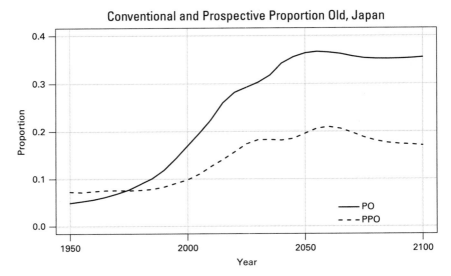

FIGURE 4.1B: Conventional and prospective proportion old, Japan. Life tables for 5-year intervals are assumed to be close approximations to life tables at the midpoints of the 5-year intervals. Populations are interpolated to the midpoints of 5-year intervals. The proportion old (PO) and the prospective proportion old (PPO) are the same in the year when remaining life expectancy at age 65 is 15 years.

Data sources: United Nations (2017c); authors' calculations.

much more substantial in the PO. At the end of the current century, the United Nations forecasts the PO to be 0.33, while the PPO is only 0.18. In other words, the PO grows almost twice as fast over the century as the PPO. So, the approach to the measurement of population aging that is adopted matters. If the onset of old age is assumed always to occur at age 65 regardless of whether we are considering 1950 or 2100, then the United Nations' forecast indicates that there would be considerable aging in Brazil's future. If the onset of old age is defined using our dynamic old-age threshold, which takes changes in life expectancy into account, we see much less aging.

As in the case of Brazil, we see in Figure 4.1b that the PO in Japan rises much more rapidly than the PPO. Both measures were similar in the early 1970s but according to United Nations' forecasts, half a century later, the PO in Japan will be almost twice as high as the PPO. It is interesting to note that, after 2065, both the PO and PPO decrease,

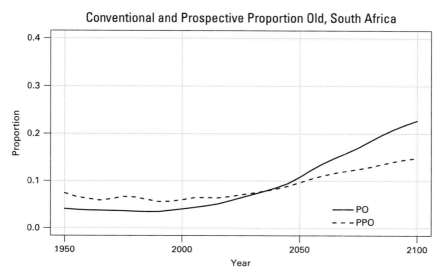

FIGURE 4.1C: Conventional and prospective proportion old, South Africa. Life tables for 5-year intervals are assumed to be close approximations to life tables at the midpoints of the 5-year intervals. Populations are interpolated to the midpoints of 5-year intervals. The proportion old (PO) and the prospective proportion old (PPO) are the same in the year when remaining life expectancy at age 65 is 15 years.

Data sources: United Nations (2017c); authors' calculations.

indicating that those measures show that Japan's population is expected to grow younger after 2065. The PPO falls more than the PO and, by the end of the century, the PPO is back to its level forecasted for the early 2020s.

The pattern of population aging looks different in South Africa depending on whether we view it using the PO or the PPO. The PO was at 0.04 in 1950 and almost triples to 0.11 by 2050. In contrast, the PPO was 0.07 in 1950 and stays around that level until 2015. The PPO then begins a slow rise, increasing to 0.10 in 2050 and to 0.15 by the end of the century.

We could produce figures like those for Brazil, Japan, and South Africa for almost all countries in the world and we would see the same results. Everywhere we look using our new glasses, we have a more realistic view of population aging.

Old-Age Dependency Ratio and
Prospective Old-Age Dependency Ratio

The OADR is one of the most commonly used age structure measures. It is the ratio of the number of adults classified as being dependent to the number of adults who could support those dependents. Adults in need of support and those who could potentially provide support can be defined in different ways (see Chapter 1). Today, the conventional approach usually assumes everyone 65 years old and older is an adult dependent and everyone from 20 to 64 is a potential provider of support. Slightly different variants of the OADR exist with different age boundaries. The United Nations publishes 5 versions of the OADR, with the beginning of support capability at ages 15, 20, or 25, and old-age dependency beginning at 65 or 70.

Does it matter whether the threshold of old-age dependency is set at a constant value of 65 (or some other fixed number) or whether it can vary according to life expectancy? To answer this question, we propose the POADR, where the stage of old age is assumed to begin at the prospective old-age threshold, instead of at age 65. This ratio varies across countries and time periods. Figures 4.2a, b, and c show the OADR and the POADR for Brazil, Japan, and South Africa. The graphs look much like those for the proportions of the population that are old in Figures 4.1a, b, and c, so we present them in a slightly different form, with values of the 2 ratios set equal to 1 in 2015. Presenting them in this way allows us to see more easily the values of the OADR and POADR relative to those in 2015.

We see in all three graphs that the POADR rises less rapidly over time than the OADR. In Brazil, in 2100, the OADR is over 5.3 times higher than it was in 2015. The increase in the POADR is substantial but not as large. At the end of the century, it is almost 3.5 times higher than its 2015 level.

Japan already has a relatively old population. Neither its OADR or its POADR is expected to increase nearly by the same percentage as in Brazil. Japan's OADR is expected to increase by around 70 percent from its 2015 level by midcentury and then stop growing. Its POADR is forecasted to increase by around 60 percent by 2065 and then fall. By 2100, it is forecasted to be about 27 percent higher than in 2015. How we expect population aging to evolve hinges on which glasses we are wearing.

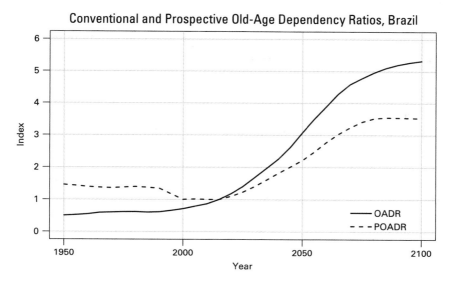

FIGURE 4.2A: Old-age dependency ratio (OADR) and prospective old-age dependency ratio (POADR), Brazil. The conventional and the prospective old-age dependency ratios are both set to 1 in 2015.

Data sources: United Nations (2017c); authors' calculations.

Using our new glasses, we can also see population aging in South Africa differently. The time path of the POADR there has a U shape. In 1950, it was around 40 percent higher than its subsequent value in 2015. The value of the POADR in the middle of the twenty-first century was about the same as it was in the middle of the twentieth century. The OADR, in contrast, is over twice as high in 2050 as it was in 1950.

Using the old glasses, we see conventional OADRs like those in Figures 4.2a, b, and c. The question that we had was whether the new glasses provided a very different vision or whether we could see the same things with the old glasses by just squinting a bit. Figures 4.2a, b, and c show that the POADRs are so different from the conventional ones that squinting will not work.

Median Age and Prospective Median Age

The change in the MA of a population is a commonly used measure of population aging. The MA of a population is defined as the age at which

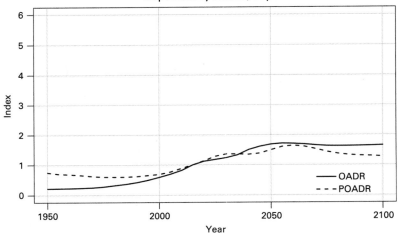

FIGURE 4.2B: Old-age dependency ratio (OADR) and prospective old-age dependency ratio (POADR), Japan. The conventional and the prospective old-age dependency ratios are both set to 1 in 2015.

Data sources: United Nations (2017c); authors' calculations.

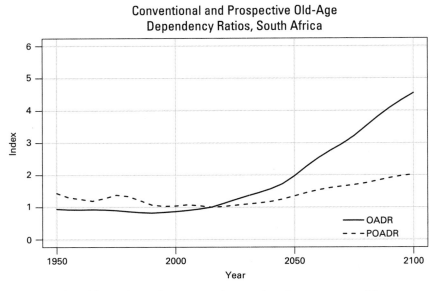

FIGURE 4.2C: Old-age dependency ratio (OADR) and prospective old-age dependency ratio (POADR), South Africa. The conventional and the prospective old-age dependency ratios are both set to 1 in 2015.

Data sources: United Nations (2017c); authors' calculations.

half the people in the population are older and half younger. In Figure 4.3a, b, and c, we present the MAs and the PMAs of the Brazilian, Japanese, and South African populations from 1950 to 2100. The PMA is the prospective age of people at the MA of the population. We can use the life expectancy schedule for any country and time period as the standard. In this section, we focus on patterns of aging in individual countries and take as standard life tables the life tables of the countries in 2010–2015. We did this because the 2010–2015 United Nations' life tables were the latest ones that the United Nations had estimated at the time we wrote this. We could have selected a life expectancy schedule from another specific year in the history of the country as a standard and observed the same general patterns. If we wanted to do a comparative study of a group of countries, we would have selected a common standard because this would have allowed us to see country differences more clearly.

For example, if the PMA of a population is 40 it means that at the MA of the population, the remaining life expectancy is the same as that of a 40-year-old person in that country in 2010–2015. Populations with the same PMA have the same remaining life expectancy at their MA. If the PMA decreases over time, it means that life expectancy at the MA is increasing over time.

Figure 4.3a shows that, in 1950, the MA of the Brazilian population was 19 years. Its PMA was around 33 years. In other words, 19-year-old Brazilians in 1950 had the same remaining life expectancy as 33-year-old Brazilians in 2015. The MA in Brazil increased from 19 in 1950–1955 to 31.3 in 2015. Did this indicate a rapid aging of the Brazilian population? Not if aging is assessed using the PMA. The PMA was around 32 in 2015. This indicates that 32-year-old Brazilians in 2015 had, on average, about the same number of remaining years to live as 19-year-old Brazilians in 1950. Over the entire period from 1950 to 2100, the MA in Brazil increases from 19 years to 50.8 years, an increase of 31.8 years. In contrast, because of increases in life expectancy, the PMA increases by only 6.5 years.

Figure 4.3b shows the paths of the MA and the PMA of the Japanese population. The increase in the PMA is much slower than in the MA. Indeed, from 2040 to the end of the century, the PMA falls. Using this measure of population aging, Japan's population would be growing younger, not older, during that period.

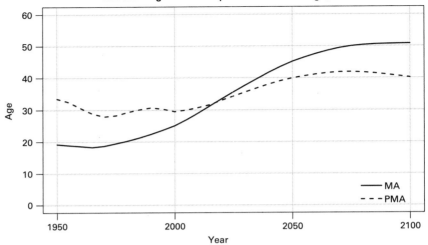

FIGURE 4.3A: Median ages (MAs) and the prospective median ages (PMAs), Brazil. The PMA is computed as the prospective age of people at the MA of the population. The computation of the PMA uses Brazil in 2010–2015 (both sexes) as the standard.

Data sources: United Nations (2017c); authors' calculations.

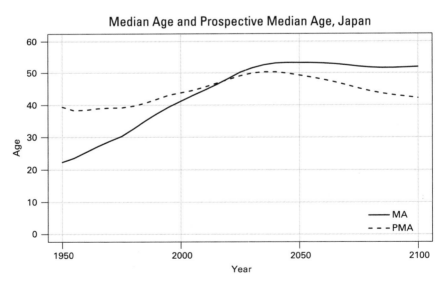

FIGURE 4.3B: Median ages (MAs) and the prospective median ages (PMAs), Japan. The PMA is computed as the prospective age of people at the MA of the population. The computation of the PMA uses Japan in 2010–2015 (both sexes) as the standard.

Data sources: United Nations (2017c); authors' calculations.

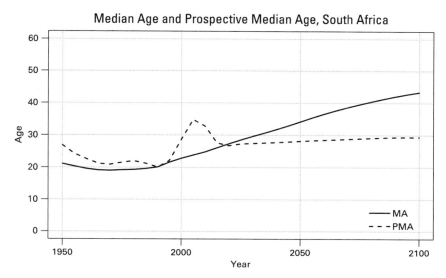

FIGURE 4.3C: Median ages (MAs) and the prospective median ages (PMAs), South Africa. The PMA is computed as the prospective age of people at the MA of the population. The computation of the PMA uses South Africa in 2010–2015 (both sexes) as the standard.

Data sources: United Nations (2017c); authors' calculations.

Figure 4.3c shows the effects of the HIV epidemic in South Africa. The MA of the South African population decreased slightly from the 1950s to the early 1970s and then rises steadily to the end of the twenty-first century. The PMA falls in the 1950s and continues to decrease until the late 1980s, when the HIV epidemic hit South Africa particularly hard. The dramatic rise in the PMA from the mid-1980s to around 2008 was due to the decrease in life expectancy caused by the disease. After the late 2000s, the PMA falls as antiretroviral treatments begin to be rolled out. After the 2030s, the PMA of the South African population stabilizes as life expectancy increases and the effect of HIV is assumed to diminish (United Nations 2017a). Again, we see that how we perceive population aging depends on which glasses we are wearing.

Proportions of 65-Year-Old Populations Who Are Old

With our new glasses we can explore parts of the demographic environment that were previously invisible. When we were wearing our old, one-dimensional glasses, everyone 65 years old or more appeared old. We could not explore the proportion of 65-year-old or older people who were old, because they all appeared that way.

If people are not automatically counted as old once they reach their 65th birthdays, then what proportion of them should be counted as old? Given the prospective old-age threshold, it is easy to answer this question. It is the ratio of the number of people who are 65 years old or older and at or above the prospective old-age threshold to those who are 65 years old or older. We present these ratios in Figures 4.4a, b, c, and d.

The proportion of the population that is 65 years old or older and above the prospective old-age threshold depends on the interaction of two aspects of population aging. First, it depends on the age structure of the population that is 65 and older. Other things equal, if a greater proportion of the 65-and-older population is 80 years old or older, for example, the proportion of the 65-and-older population who are old will be higher. Second, it also depends on the prospective old-age threshold. Other things being constant, the higher the prospective old-age threshold, the lower the proportion of the 65-and-older population whom we would count as old.

In Figure 4.4a, we compare the proportion of people 65 years old and older in Brazil and Chile who would be counted as old, using the prospective old-age threshold. In 1950, 100 percent of 65-year-old and older people in both countries would be above the old-age threshold because remaining life expectancy at age 65 was below 15 years in both. Remaining life expectancy first rises above 15 years at age 65 in 2000 in Brazil and more than a decade earlier in Chile. By 2015, the proportion of 65-year-olds who we would classify as old fell to 64 percent in Brazil and 59 percent in Chile. Viewing the onset of old age from the perspective of how many years people have left to live instead of how many years they have already lived makes a substantial difference. After 2030, the proportions of people 65 and older who are old roughly stabilizes in both countries. In Brazil that proportion stays near 55 percent. In Chile, it roughly stabilizes at 51 percent.

In Figure 4.4b, we compare China and India. In China, life expectancy at age 65 rises above 15 years in 2005. The United Nations forecasts this to occur in India in 2030. The proportions of the 65-and-older population who are old fall in both countries, reaching 71 percent and

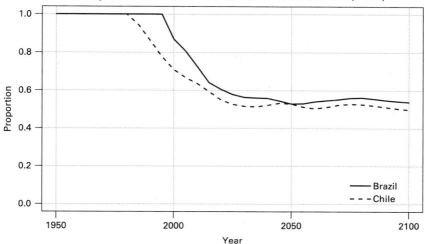

FIGURE 4.4A: Proportion of population 65 and older who are old (P65O), Brazil and Chile. Proportions of populations 65 years old and older who are counted as being old are the proportions of those populations who are at or older than the prospective old-age threshold.

Data sources: United Nations (2017c); authors' calculations.

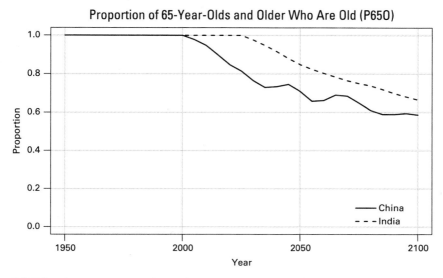

FIGURE 4.4B: Proportion of population 65 and older who are old, China and India (P65O). Proportions of populations 65 years old and older who are counted as being old are the proportions of those populations who are at or older than the prospective old-age threshold.

Data sources: United Nations (2017c); authors' calculations.

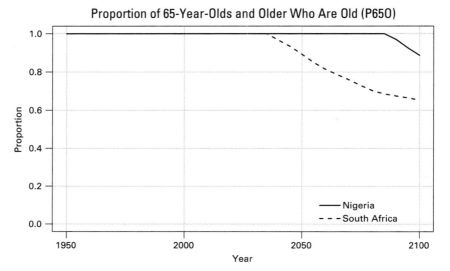

FIGURE 4.4C: Proportion of population 65 and older who are old (P65O), Nigeria and South Africa. Proportions of populations 65 years old and older who are counted as being old are the proportions of those populations who are at or older than the prospective old-age threshold.

Data sources: United Nations (2017c); authors' calculations.

85 percent, respectively, in China and India in 2050. In the second half of the century, the proportions of the 65-and-older populations who are old move downward to 59 percent in China and 67 percent in India by 2100.

In Figure 4.4c, we compare Nigeria and South Africa. The United Nations forecasts life expectancy at age 65 to first rise above 15 years in Nigeria in 2090, so the proportion of the 65-and-older Nigerians that we would classify as being old remains at 100 percent until then. In South Africa, life expectancy at 65 is forecasted to rise above 15 years in 2040. After that, the proportion of those aged 65 and older who are old falls to 65 percent by the end of the century.

In Figure 4.4d, we compare Japan, the Russian Federation, and the United States. In Japan, life expectancy at age 65 rose above 15 years in 1978. In the Russian Federation, this occurred in 2015 and in the United States in 1975. By 2015, only 55 percent of Japanese above age 65 would be

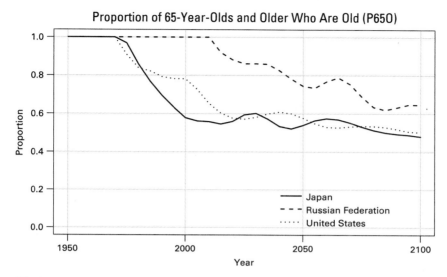

FIGURE 4.4D: Proportion of population 65 and older who are old (P65O), Japan, Russia, and United States. Proportions of populations 65 years old and older who are counted as being old are the proportions of those populations who are at or older than the prospective old-age threshold.

Data sources: United Nations (2017c); authors' calculations.

classified as old and only 60 percent of the Americans. For the remainder of the century, that proportion falls slowly in both countries, reaching 65 percent in Japan by 2100 and 50 percent in the United States. In the Russian Federation, it falls to 65 percent by the end of the century.

When we have only one-dimensional vision, everyone everywhere looks old at age 65. When we have two-dimensional vision, we can separate who is old from who is 65 years old and older. This separation is an interesting new feature of the demographic environment that we can now see with our new glasses.

Conclusion

There was a time when the sole characteristic of people used in measures of population aging was their chronological age. Now, this is no longer the case. With our new glasses, when we look at familiar measures of population aging, like the OADR and the MA, we see things differently. But perhaps even more exciting, we can see things like the proportion of people 65 years old and older who are old (according to the prospective old-age threshold). There is no measure like this in the one-dimensional world.

4

Note on NTA Economic Support Ratio

Before the *prospective old-age dependency ratio (POADR)* appeared in United Nations (2017b), the newest measure of population aging used by the United Nations Population Division was the *economic support ratio* (United Nations 2015) produced by the National Transfer Accounts project (NTA, n.d.a). The NTA project is a large and productive international undertaking that combines economics and demography. The project has taken standard economic aggregates and transformed them into age-specific magnitudes. The numerator of the economic support ratio adds people of all ages together based on production weights and the denominator does the same using consumption weights. The resulting ratio has two important features. First, the production and consumption weights are observations that are country and time specific. For example, the NTA website, at this writing (November 2017), provides consumption and production weights for 59 countries, including Côte d'Ivoire in 2015, India in 2004, China in 2007, the United States in 2011, Austria in 2010, Germany in 2008, Brazil in 2002, and Mexico in 2010 (NTA, n.d.a). The second feature is that the NTA economic support ratio does not use an old-age threshold and, therefore, does not categorize people as old.

From our perspective, the chief difficulty with using NTA support ratios for analyzing population aging in the future is that the age-specific production and consumption weights are influenced by economic conditions and policies that could change quickly over time. Barslund and Werder (2017) tackle this problem. They create a new type of NTA economic support ratio based on age-specific transfers, which they allow to vary over time with health, migration, and length of working life. They show that allowing or not allowing these types of time variation in age-specific transfers matters, but data limitations kept them from studying more than a handful of countries.

There are many potential synergies between the NTA approach and ours. We look forward one day to the existence of a set of prospective economic support ratios.

5

Determining Ages Based on the Characteristics of People

WHEN YOU STEP out of a dark room into bright sunlight, it takes a moment for your eyes to adjust. But when people have learned about age and aging from a single perspective all their lives, it could take more than a moment to adjust to being able to see things more clearly. "How old are you?" will always mean how many birthdays have you had. But how many birthdays people have celebrated is only one piece of information. People of the same age in different countries, at different times, and in different educational groups are not all the same. Being blind to these differences is akin to living in a very dimly lit room. In the preceding chapters, we have opened the door halfway so that an important aspect of people's lives, how long they have yet to live, could illuminate the surroundings. When we did so, population aging could be seen more clearly. Now that you have had some time to adjust, we open the door all the way.

In this chapter, we broaden our view of population aging, allowing it to encompass characteristics of people in addition to remaining life expectancy. In doing this, two related problems immediately arise. First, characteristics related to population aging are quantified using different metrics. Hand-grip strength, for example, is a measure of upper body strength related to future mortality and morbidity (Sanderson and Scherbov 2014; Sanderson et al. 2016; Hanten et al. 1999; Al Snih et al. 2004; Bohannon 2001; Fukumori et al. 2015; Koopman et al.

2015; Ling et al. 2010; Cooper et al. 2014; Roberts et al. 2011). It is generally measured in kilograms. Further, a commonly used test of cognition is the delayed word recall test, where people are asked to recall a series of words stated earlier in an interview (Anstey et al. 2001; Bordone, Scherbov, and Steiber 2015; Skirbekk, Loichinger, and Weber 2012; Weber et al. 2014). The score on that test is the number of words correctly remembered. Thus, as soon as we think about population aging in a multidimensional framework, we encounter the problem of incommensurate measures that are difficult to relate to one another.

The second problem magnifies the first. Not only are many characteristics of people measured in different units, exactly how characteristics are related to aging is often unclear. For example, should the relationship between age and hand-grip strength be expressed in terms of number of kilograms or the square root of the number of kilograms? The probability of surviving for the subsequent 5 years and the probability of dying within that period are two ways of measuring the same thing. New measures of aging should be the same regardless of whether hand-grip strength is expressed in terms of kilograms or the square root of that number or whether mortality conditions are expressed in terms of death rates or survival rates.

The challenge, then, is clear. It is to take measures, as different as hand-grip strength, the number of words recalled, disability rates, and self-rated health, and study them within a clear, consistent, and informative framework.

Fortunately, a simple generalization of the measures of aging that we have already discussed in Chapter 2 is all that is needed. In that chapter, we distinguished two ways of computing ages based on the characteristics of people. One was to produce ages based on a fixed remaining life expectancy. We called these *prospective constant characteristic ages.* The other was to compute the prospective age associated with a chronological age. That prospective age was the age in a *standard population* where people had the same level of remaining life expectancy as at the specified chronological age. In this chapter, we show that the new glasses allow full multidimensional vision by demonstrating that characteristic-based ages, analogous to prospective ages and prospective constant characteristic ages, can be computed using many characteristics of people in addition to their remaining life expectancy.

Constant Characteristic Ages

Constant characteristic ages are ages in different populations where the level of a characteristic is constant. The *prospective old-age threshold*, discussed in Chapter 3, is an example of a constant characteristic age. The characteristic is remaining life expectancy and its constant level is 15 years. Another example of the determination of constant characteristic ages is shown in Table 5.1.

The hypothetical characteristic values in Table 5.1 are average hand-grip strengths. The fixed characteristic level, k_1, is an average hand-grip strength of 30 kilograms. We see that 57-year-olds in 1950 had an average hand-grip strength of 30 kilograms (a_1), that 60-year-olds in 1975 had the same average hand-grip strength (a_2), as well as 63-year-olds in 2000 (a_3). The ages 57 in 1950, 60 in 1975, and 63 in 2000 are all constant characteristic ages because people at those ages had the same average hand-grip strength (30 kilograms).

Table 5.2 provides another example, this one is based roughly on the life tables of Canadian women in the Human Mortality Database (University of California, Berkeley, and Max Planck Institute for Demographic Research 2017).

In Table 5.2, the fixed characteristic is a 2 percent chance of dying within 1 year of the indicated age (k_1). In 1950, that was the probability of dying experienced by 64-year-old Canadian women (a_1). In 1975, the same probability of dying was experienced by 69-year-old Canadian women (a_2) and in 2000 by 73-year-old Canadian women (a_3). Therefore, when we choose a characteristic level of a 2 percent chance of

Table 5.1 Constant characteristic ages, average hand-grip strength, hypothetical values

k_1	a_1	k_1	a_2	k_1	a_3
Average hand-grip strength	Age in 1950 with the indicated hand-grip strength	Average hand-grip strength	Age in 1975 with the indicated hand-grip strength	Average hand-grip strength	Age in 2000 with the indicated hand-grip strength
30 kg	57	**30 kg**	60	**30 kg**	63

Table 5.2 Constant characteristic ages, annual probability of dying within
1 year, Canadian women

k_1	a_1	k_1	a_2	k_1	a_3
Annual probability of dying	Age in 1950 with the indicated probability	Annual probability of dying	Age in 1975 with the indicated probability	Annual probability of dying	Age in 2000 with the indicated probability
2 percent	64	**2 percent**	69	**2 percent**	73

Data source: University of California, Berkeley, and Max Planck Institute for
Demographic Research (2017).

dying within the coming year, 64-year-old Canadian women in 1950,
69-year-old Canadian women in 1975, and 73-year-old Canadian women
in 2000 all have the same constant characteristic age.

In Table 5.1, we translated hand-grip strengths into constant characteristic ages, and, in Table 5.2, we translated annual probabilities of
dying into constant characteristic ages. The same sort of translation
can be done for a wide variety of characteristics and because the results are in terms of ages, they can be compared and analyzed within
a consistent framework.

α-Ages

In Chapter 2, we discussed the computation of prospective ages associated with specific chronological ages. Those ages were ages in a standard population where people had the same levels of remaining life
expectancy as at the specific chronological ages. When this approach
is generalized, we obtain what we call *α-ages*. Instead of starting with
a characteristic level, as we do when we compute constant characteristic ages, the computation of α-ages starts with a chronological age.
For example, that age might be 70; and 70-year-old people in different
countries, in different times, and in different subgroups are likely to
have different levels of characteristics germane to the study of population aging. If all we can see is that these people are 70 years old, we
would be blind to important ways in which they differ from one another. In order to improve our vision of 70-year-olds, we need a method

of quantifying their differences which can be applied consistently across a variety of characteristics. α-ages allow us to look over time and space and see how people of the same chronological age differ from one another. A 70-year-old person in one country might have an α-age of 72 based on one characteristic and 71 based on another, even though those characteristics are measured in different units. A 70-year-old person in another country could have an α-age of 68 based on the first characteristic and 69 based on the second one. α-ages permit a new multidimensional view of population aging, one based on the translation of multiple characteristics into the common metric of age.

We provide a hypothetical example of the computation of α-ages in Tables 5.3a and 5.3b. Imagine that we had data on the relationship between average hand-grip strength and age for women in a specific country in 1950 and 2000. Average hand-grip strength is an indicator of upper body strength and a good predictor of subsequent mortality and morbidity, so it is pertinent to the study of population aging. In Table 5.3a, we assume that the average hand-grip strength of 65-year-old women in 1950 (a) was 30 kilograms (k_1). To find the α-age of those women, we need to find the age in the standard characteristic schedule where women had an average hand-grip strength of 30 kilograms. In Table 5.3a, the standard characteristic schedule is the relationship between average hand-grip strength and age in the country's population in the year 2000. In the hypothetical example, in Table 5.3a, that age would be 72. So, the α-age of 65-year-old women in the hypothetical country in 1950 would be 72, using the characteristic schedule of 2000 as the standard of comparison.

In Table 5.3b, we follow the same steps using the 1-year probability of dying as the characteristic. We again begin with 65-year-old women in our hypothetical country (a) and see that the probability of them dying in 1950 was 0.02 (k_1). When we use the life table for 2000 in that country and the standard, we see that 75-year-old women in that year have the same 1-year probability of dying. Therefore, the α-age of the 65-year-old women was 75 when we use the characteristic schedule of 2000 as the standard.

Tables 5.3a and 5.3b show how two different characteristics of women can be quantified using α-ages. The tables show that the α-age of 65-year-old women using hand-grip strength as the characteristic was

Table 5.3a   Computation of the α-age for 65-year-olds in 1950, using the 2000 characteristic schedule as the standard

a	k1	k1	α-age
Chronological age in 1950	Hand-grip strength in 1950 at the indicated chronological age (in kg)	Hand-grip strength in 2000 (standard) (in kg)	α-age (age in 2000) where hand-grip strength is what it was at the chronological age in 1950
65	30	30	72

Table 5.3b   Computation of the α-age for 65-year-old women in 1950, using 2000 as the standard

age (a)	k1	k1	α-age
Chronological age in 1950	Probability of dying within 1 year at the indicated chronological age in 1950	Probability of dying within 1 year in 2000 (standard)	α-age (age in 2000) where 1-year death rate is what it was at the chronological age in 1950
65	0.02	0.02	75

lower than the one obtained using the 1-year survival rate, and, therefore, that the women aged more rapidly in terms of upper-body strength (as measured by hand-grip strength) than they did in terms of their 1-year survival rate.

Comparing Constant Characteristic Ages Based on Life Table Characteristics

The most commonly used life table characteristic in the study of population aging is life expectancy. Survival or death rates rank a distant second, and one of the most interesting life table–based characteristics has rarely been used. That characteristic is the proportion of adult lifetimes lived after various ages. For example, in some places people might spend 10 percent of their adult lifetimes over 65 years old. In other places, it might be 25 percent. Demographers compute proportions of adult lifetimes lived after various ages using the concept of person-years.

In Table 5.4, we show an example of how the proportion of adult lifetimes lived after the age of 75 can be computed. The population in that table consists of ten people. In the middle column, we have the number of years each person lives from his or her 20th birthday onward. Person 1, for example, lived 66.4 years after age 20, or, in other words, she died at age 86.4. The total number of person-years lived by all people in the population is obtained by summing the middle column. The ten people in the population lived a total of 600 person-years and the average number of person-years lived by the ten people in the population is 60. The average number of person-years lived by people in a population beginning at a specific age is their remaining life expectancy at that age. So, the remaining life expectancy at age 20 of our ten-person population is 60 years.

The right column shows the number of person-years lived from age 75 onward. Person 1 lived to age 86.4, so she lived 11.4 years after her 75th birthday. Person 2 died at age 32.7, so did not reach his 75th birthday. Summing all the person-years lived from age 75 onward among the ten people in our population, we see that they lived 75.1 person-years. The ten people in the population lived a total of 600 years from age 20 onward of which 75.1 of those years were lived at age 75 or above. Therefore, the fraction of all the years lived from age 20 onward that were also lived from age 75 onward is 75.1 divided by 600 or 0.125. Put differently, in this example, one-eighth of the adult lifetime is spent at age 75 or above.

Demographers use the notation T_x to refer to the total number of *person-years lived from age x onward*. Therefore, T_{75}/T_{20} is equal to 0.125 (75.1 divided by 600). We call these ratios *life course ratios at age x* (or simply *life course ratios*) and they are the fraction of adult person-years lived from age x onward.

Life course ratios are an interesting aspect of populations to observe when studying aging. While they are used far less frequently than life

Table 5.4 Example of the computation of the number of adult
person-years lived by a population of ten people and the
number of person-years that they lived from age 75 and onward

Person	Number of years lived from age 20 onward	Number of years lived from age 75 onward
1	66.4	11.4
2	32.7	0
3	52.2	0
4	68.9	13.9
5	72.8	17.8
6	59.7	4.7
7	63.5	8.5
8	61.2	6.2
9	59.8	4.8
10	62.8	7.8
Total	600	75.1

expectancies, they are, nevertheless, very informative. We use them in Chapter 6 to discuss what fraction of the adult lifetime is spent in old age, and, in Chapter 12, to derive *intergenerationally equitable normal pension ages*.

In Figure 5.1, we present graphical examples of how characteristic ages using the life course ratio are determined using three characteristic schedules: those for Japan, the Russian Federation, and the United States in 2010. The characteristic schedules are taken from the Human Mortality Database. A horizontal line is drawn at a life course ratio of 0.25. The ages where people have this level of characteristic are the ages where 25 percent of all adult person-years in the life table are yet to be lived. In the Russian Federation, that constant characteristic age was 57.3. In the United States, it was 65.4 and in Japan it was 66.6.

One application of constant characteristic ages is in the field of public policy. Shoven and Goda (2010) used four life table characteristics and computed how the associated chronological ages would have changed if various pieces of US legislation had been written in terms of those characteristics instead of chronological age. Those characteristics were a constant remaining life expectancy, a constant death rate, a constant percentage of life expectancy at birth, and a constant percentage of life expectancy at age 20. The legislation

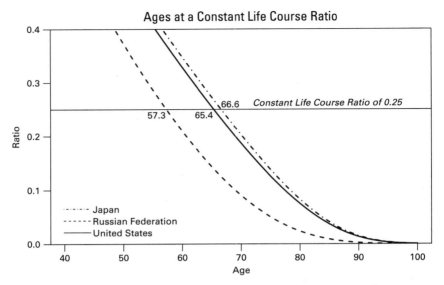

FIGURE 5.1: Constant characteristic ages for Japan, the Russian Federation, and the United States for 2010, based on life course ratios.

Data source: University of California, Berkeley, and Max Planck Institute for Demographic Research (2017).

studied included the normal social security pension age, the age eligibility for Medicare (health insurance), and aspects of individual retirement accounts.

The work of Shoven and Goda challenges policymakers with an important question: Should public policies be formulated based on fixed chronological ages or some characteristic of people that changes over time? Their research clearly demonstrates that it makes a substantial difference which approach is used. Implicitly, their paper also raises one of the greatest difficulties with this approach. It is not clear which constant characteristic age is appropriate for which policy. The application of constant characteristic ages to public policies requires a clear answer to this question. Fortunately, with our new glasses, we can see how this question should be answered for normal public pension ages. In Chapter 12, we show that the answer does not involve any of the four characteristics used in Shoven and Goda (2010) but rather the life course ratio.

Comparing α-Ages Based on Life Table Characteristics

In Figure 5.2, we present the same three characteristic schedules as in Figure 5.1 and, instead of showing how constant characteristic ages are computed, we show the derivation of α-ages. To do this, we draw a vertical line at age 65 and designate the characteristic schedule for the United States as the standard. We see that the α-age of 65-year-old Japanese in 2010 was 63.7, using the United States characteristic schedule in 2010 as the standard. The α-age of 65-year-old Russians in 2010 was 73.5, using the same standard schedule. In 2010, 65-year-old Russians had the same portion of their adult person-years ahead of them as 73.5-year-old Americans in the same year.

In Figures 5.3 and 5.4, we illustrate the evolution of constant characteristic ages and α-ages for Australia, England and Wales, France, Sweden, Switzerland, and the United States using three characteristics: (1) remaining life expectancy, (2) the 5-year mortality rate, and (3) the

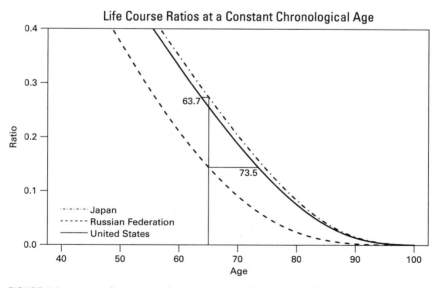

FIGURE 5.2: α-ages for Japan, the Russian Federation, and the United States for 2010. The characteristic is the life course ratio, US population in 2010 as standard schedule.

Data source: University of California, Berkeley, and Max Planck Institute for Demographic Research (2017).

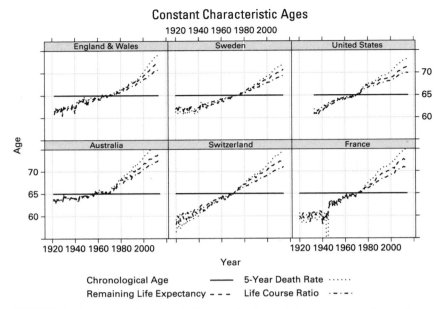

Constant Characteristic Ages

FIGURE 5.3: Constant characteristic ages for four characteristics, chronological age, remaining life expectancy, the 5-year survival rate and the life course ratio in Australia, England and Wales, France, Sweden, Switzerland, and the United States, 1920 to 2010. The 1970 characteristic schedules for each country are used as the standards.

Data sources: University of California, Berkeley, and Max Planck Institute for Demographic Research (2017); authors' calculations.

life course ratio as well as chronological age. In Figure 5.3, constant characteristic ages are plotted assuming that for each country the constant characteristic levels are the values observed for 65-year-olds in 1970. Because of this assumption, the constant characteristic ages for all three characteristics were 65 in 1970.

We see that, over time, the constant characteristic ages generally increase, reflecting the effects of increases in survival rates. As life expectancy increases, the same remaining life expectancy observed for 65-year-olds in 1970 is observed at progressively older ages. For all six countries, the same remaining life expectancy that was observed for 65-year-olds in 1970 was observed above age 70 in 2010. The speed of increase is not the same for the three different characteristics. The con-

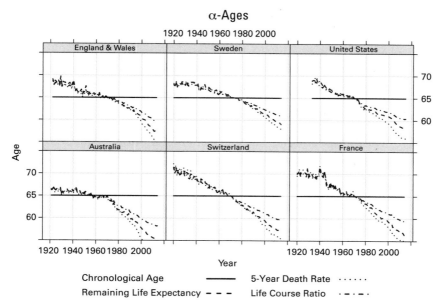

FIGURE 5.4: α-ages for four characteristics, chronological age, remaining life expectancy, the 5-year survival rate and the life course ratio, in Australia, England and Wales, France, Sweden, Switzerland, and the United States, 1920 to 2010. The 1970 characteristic schedules for each country are used as the standards.

Data sources: University of California, Berkeley, and Max Planck Institute for Demographic Research (2017); authors' calculations.

stant characteristic age for the 5-year mortality rate increases the fastest, followed by the constant characteristic age based on remaining life expectancy. The constant characteristic age based on the life course ratio increases most slowly. We discuss some of the implications of this in Chapter 6.

Figure 5.4 shows the evolution of α-ages for the same six countries over the same time period. α-ages are plotted for 65-year-olds in various years, using the characteristic schedules in each country in 1970 as standards. This construction guarantees that all the α-ages in 1970 are 65. We see a general downward trend in the α-ages. This means that as mortality conditions improve, the characteristic levels observed for 65-year-olds would be the same as those in the 1970 standard population at progressively earlier ages. We also see that the speed at which the α-ages change over time differs depending on which characteristic is considered. The α-age graphs based on the 5-year mortality rate fall most rapidly and the ones for the life course ratio fall the slowest.

Comparing Survey-Based Characteristics

Surveys on aging are a rich source of characteristic schedules that can be used to compute α-ages. In Sanderson et al. (2016), we used α-ages to study differences across educational subgroups in hand-grip strength and chair-rise speed, as well as how well they predicted subgroup differences in survival in England. The two subgroups were those with more education (high school graduation or equivalent or beyond, NVQ 2, GCE, or higher) and those with less education (less than high school graduation, no qualification, NVQ 1, or CSE).

Using data from the 2004 wave of the English Longitudinal Study of Ageing (ELSA), we computed the differences between α-ages and chronological ages for hand-grip strength and chair-rise speed for the more educated subgroup using the characteristic schedules of the less educated as standards.

Differences between α-ages and chronological ages quantify the advantage or disadvantage that one subgroup has relative to the other. Using data from the 2004 and 2012 waves of the survey, we also computed the differences between α-ages and chronological ages based on survival.

In Table 5.5, we provide an example of how combining information about two different characteristics of people can be done. All the numbers in the table are negative. Women with more education had the same average hand-grip strength as less educated women who were 4.0 years younger. Women with more education had the same chair-rise speed as women with less education who were 3.2 years younger. Although hand-grip strength and chair-rise speed are measured in different units, here, they are both translated into the same units, years of age, so we can take their average. The average age difference is −3.6 years. When we computed the age difference using the survival rate from 2004 to 2012, we found that women with more education had the same 8-year survival rates as less educated women 3.6 years younger.

Table 5.5 Difference between α-ages and chronological ages for people with more education using the characteristic schedules for people with less education as the standards: ages 60–85

Characteristic	Women	Men
Hand-grip strength, 2004	−4.0	−3.5
Chair-rise speed, 2004	−3.2	−5.2
Average	−3.6	−4.4
Survival, 2004–2012	−3.6	−4.1

Data source: Sanderson et al. (2016, table 10).

Note: Differences between α-ages and chronological ages were invariant in the age range 60–85.

So, for women, the average of the age differences based on two physical tests in 2004, predicted the age difference in subsequent survival perfectly. For men, the average did not predict quite as well, but still better than either hand-grip strength or chair-rise speed taken separately. Table 5.5 illustrates an important feature of α-ages. Quantities based on α-ages are in the same units, so that it is possible to combine them by taking averages or using other statistics.

Surveys provide a rich source of information on population aging. Translating these characteristics into α-ages so that they are expressed in a common unit, as in the example in Table 5.5, allows us to see population aging from a fully multidimensional perspective.

Conclusion

We have many megabytes of constant characteristic ages and α-ages on our computers, far more than we have space for here. Constant characteristic ages and α-ages are the lens through which we view population aging. So, let us continue our exploration of the demographic environment in the following chapters. With our new glasses, aspects of population aging will now be in sharper focus and we will be less likely to lose our way.

5

Mathematical Appendix

The fundamental building block in the computation of *constant characteristic ages* and *α-ages* is a *characteristic schedule*, $C_r(a)$. The schedule relates chronological age a to some value, k, of a characteristic in population r, called the index population

$$k = C_r(a). \tag{5.A1}$$

For example, the characteristic schedule could relate chronological age to the average hand-grip strength of people of chronological age a in population r, to the square root of the average hand-grip strength or to any monotonic transformation of the average hand-grip strength. The schedule $C_r(a)$ must be monotonic and continuous over an appropriate range of ages. Details about the range of ages over which $C_r(a)$ is defined are discussed below.

In this case, $C_r(a)$ is invertible, so that we can write

$$a = C_r^{-1}(k). \tag{5.A2}$$

Given a set of characteristic schedules $(r_1, r_2, \ldots, r_n)$ and a characteristic level k, equation (5.A2) produces a corresponding set of constant characteristic ages $(a_1, a_2, \ldots, a_n)$.

Constant characteristic ages do not require a *standard schedule* but, to compute α-ages, one is needed. Let us denote the standard schedule using the subscript s. α-ages are ages in the standard schedule where people have the same value of the characteristic as they have at a particular age in the index population, r, so we can write

$$\alpha = C_s^{-1}(k). \tag{5.A3}$$

Equation (5.A3) computes an α-age, the chronological age in the standard population, where people have a specified value of the characteristic.

Substituting equation (5.A1) into (5.A3), we obtain

$$\alpha_{a,r,s} = C_s^{-1}[C_r(a)] \tag{5.A4}$$

where $\alpha_{a,r,s}$ is the α-age associated with chronological age a, in population r, using population s as a standard. The α-age, $\alpha_{a,r,s}$, depends on the chronological age of the people in the index population r, on the population, s, that is used as a standard and on the characteristic used.

Equation (5.A4) translates chronological ages into α-ages. It is also possible to translate α-ages into chronological ages:

$$a_{\alpha,r,s} = C_r^{-1}[C_s(\alpha)] \qquad (5.A5)$$

where $a_{\alpha,r,s}$ is the chronological age in index population r associated with the α-age, α, in standard population, s. Fixing α and s, equation (5.A5) is equivalent to equation (5.A2) and can be used to compute constant characteristic ages.

There are some special cases of characteristic schedules which produce relatively simple relationships between chronological ages and α-ages. To derive these, we begin with a more general formulation and then obtain specific relationships from it:

$$Q(k) = A_j + B_j \cdot g(age), \text{ where } j = (r,s). \qquad (5.A6)$$

Equation (5.A6) is a special case of equation (5.A1), $Q(k)$ is a continuous and monotonic function of characteristic k and $g(age)$ is a continuous and monotonic function of age.

Since α-ages are computed by equating the value of the characteristic in the index population and the standard population, this is the same as equating the values of $Q(k)$ in the two populations. Therefore,

$$A_s + B_s \cdot g(\alpha) = A_r + B_r \cdot g(age) \qquad (5.A7)$$

and

$$\alpha = g^{-1} \left[\frac{A_r - A_s + B_r \cdot g(age)}{B_s} \right] \qquad (5.A8)$$

One of the most important features of equation (5.A8) is that the transformation $Q(k)$ has vanished, so the equation holds for any continuous and monotonic $Q(k)$. In particular, equation 5.A8 indicates that the same α-ages would be obtained if we were studying age-specific mortality rates or age-specific survival rates.

The simplest special cases of equation (5.A8) occur when $g(age) = age$, in this case,

$$\alpha = \frac{(A_r - A_s)}{B_s} + \left(\frac{B_r}{B_s}\right) \cdot age \qquad (5.A9)$$

Whenever $g(age)=age$, equation (5.A6) also becomes

$$Q(k) = A_j + B_j \cdot age, \text{ where } j = (r,s). \qquad (5.A10)$$

Equation (5.A10) expresses the relationship between chronological age and values of characteristics for a variety of characteristic schedules. For example, the characteristic schedule could be

$$k = \frac{e^{A_j + B_j \cdot age}}{1 + e^{A_j + B_j \cdot age}}, j = (r,s). \qquad (5.A11)$$

$$\text{Setting } Q(k) = \ln\left(\frac{k}{1-k}\right), \qquad (5.A12)$$

and combining equations (5.A11) and (5.A12), yields equation (5.A10) and, therefore,

$$\alpha = \frac{(A_r - A_s)}{B_s} + \left(\frac{B_r}{B_s}\right) \cdot age. \qquad (5.A13)$$

Many characteristic functions would result in the linear relationship between chronological age and α-age that we observe in equation (5.A13), so the exact shape of the characteristic function cannot be inferred from that linearity.

Another special case of equation (5.A8) arises when $g(age) = 1/age$. In this case, the relationship between chronological and α-age is given by

$$\alpha = \frac{B_s}{A_r - A_s + B_r\left(\dfrac{1}{age}\right)}. \qquad (5.A14)$$

An additional special case of equation (5.A8) arises when $g(age) = ln(age)$. In this instance,

$$\alpha = e^{\frac{(A_r - A_s)}{B_s}} \cdot age^{\left(\frac{B_r}{B_s}\right)}. \qquad (5.A15)$$

The analytical relationships that we have derived here hint at the complexity of the possible relationships between chronological and α-ages. They can help in interpreting the relationships that we observe in the data, but we should be aware that observed relationships can be far more complex than the simple examples that we have generated here.

There are two technical problems that arise in the computation of α-ages. First, α-ages do not always exist. In this book, we are interested in the α-ages of older individuals, so the characteristic schedules need to be defined over some age range, say $[a_{min}, a_{max}]$, where a_{min} and a_{max} are the minimum and maximum chronological ages of interest. The minimum and maximum values of C_r defined over that age range are denoted $[C_{r,min}, C_{r,max}]$, respectively, and the analogous values for C_s are $[C_{s,min}, C_{s,max}]$. It is possible that there are values of the characteristic in the range $[C_{r,min}, C_{r,max}]$ that fall outside the range $[C_{s,min}, C_{s,max}]$. When the characteristic in population r has such values, α-ages cannot be computed.

The nonexistence of some α-ages is not generally a problem and can be dealt with by the appropriate choice of the standard population. One approach is to choose the standard population as the one with the highest values of the characteristic. If $C_{r,min} = C_{s,min}$ and $C_s(a) > C_r(a)$, for a in the interval $[a_{min}, a_{max}]$, then α-ages will always exist for chronological ages in the relevant range.

The second problem is subtler. Characteristic schedules can be monotonic in chronological age, but the increase or decrease in the schedule can be so small as to be practically unobservable. Although technically the characteristic does vary with age, the variation does not permit meaningful analysis. For example, if the level of some characteristic is almost the same for 40-year-olds and 60-year-olds, we cannot use that age range in the computation of α-ages.

6

The Stage of Old Age

IN EXPLORING ASPECTS of the demographic environment that we can see with the new glasses, our next stop is not a place but a life cycle stage—the stage of old age. The stage of old age is a social construct. Its primary usefulness is in practical matters. Important public policies are based on how old age is defined. We might be led to believe that old age begins when a person is eligible to receive a full public pension or perhaps at the age of mandatory retirement. Perhaps we are led to believe that old age begins when we can get discounts on public transportation, movie tickets, or when we can first order the special dishes cooked for "seniors" in restaurants. Perhaps, we are led to believe that we are old when we read newspaper articles about the misfortunes of an "elderly" woman or man who is younger than we are. In numerous, sometimes barely noticeable ways, people are influenced by the definition of old age.

In many United Nations publications, old age begins either at age 60 or 65. According to Eurostat, the US Census Bureau, and the OECD, it is 65. Among the major statistical agencies, only the World Bank admits that there is some ambiguity about the number (World Bank 2016; Bussolo, Koettl, and Sinnott 2015). Hundreds of academic books and articles, newspaper articles, and websites tell us that people should be categorized as old at age 65.

From Ballod (1913) onward (see Chapter 1), one of the major conceptualizations of old age has been as a period of dependency and burden.

The natural question in that context is how much of a burden the elderly will be on those who support them. In this chapter and Chapter 7, we take a different approach and focus on aspects of the period during which people are categorized as being old.

In this book, we have distinguished two views of old age. One view is that there is a fixed chronological age boundary, usually 60 or 65, and all people older than this threshold would be categorized as old regardless of country, time period, or any other characteristic. Our view is that the old-age threshold should depend on the characteristics of the group being studied. Our preferred specification of the old-age threshold is the age at which remaining life expectancy is 15 years. So, we envision two hypothetical paths from the onset of adulthood: one leading to an old-age threshold of age 65, the *conventional old-age threshold*, and another leading to the *prospective old-age threshold (POAT)*. In this chapter we analyze the fraction of the adult lifetime that is spent in old age on each of those two paths.

We use two sorts of life tables in our analysis, cohort life tables and period life tables. Up to now our computations have used period life tables because these are more numerous and up to date. Period life tables provide statistics based on the age-specific survival rates in a particular period. For example, life expectancy at age 65 in 2015 is what the average number of years 65-year-olds would have left to live using the survival rates of 2015. Cohort life tables are different from the period life tables that we have been using. They follow actual groups of people over their lifetimes. In 2015, 65-year-olds were born in 1950. The cohort life expectancy of 65-year-olds born in 1950 would need to be computed from survival rates from 2015 onward until there were few people born in 1950 still alive. Naturally, the data needed to compute that life expectancy are not currently available, but nearly complete cohort life tables are available for some countries for cohorts born in the late nineteenth and early twentieth centuries.

Proportion of Adult Lifetime in Old Age Based on Cohort Life Tables

The proportions of adult lifetimes spent beyond the conventional and prospective old-age thresholds can be computed from cohort life tables in the Human Mortality Database (HMD) (University of California, Berkeley, and Max Planck Institute for Demographic Research 2017). In Tables 6.1a and 6.1b, we compute this for nine countries: Denmark, England and Wales, Finland, France, Iceland, Italy, the Netherlands, Sweden, and Switzerland, and for cohorts born from 1860 to 1920 at 20-year intervals. Cohort life tables in the HMD are produced after 100 percent of the people born in a particular year have already died and for almost-extinct cohorts. The most recent cohort life tables in the HMD are for people born in the early 1920s.

The data in Table 6.1a are ratios of the number of *person-years lived from age 65 and onward* to all the person-years lived from age 20 and onward. For one person, the number of person-years lived from age 20 onward is the number of years the person has lived from age 20 to his death. When we look at a group of people, the number of person-years lived from age 20 onward is the sum of the individual person-years. The number of person-years lived from any age onward can be calculated in the same way.

The data in Table 6.1b are the ratios of the number of person-years lived from the POAT and onward to all the person-years lived from age 20 onward. In the terminology of Chapter 5, these ratios are *life course ratios.*

Using 65 as the old-age threshold, we see in Table 6.1a that around 17 percent of the adult person-years of the people born in 1860 were spent in old age and that this percentage increased for later-born cohorts. People born in 1920 would have spent around one-quarter of their adult person-years in old age. Using age 65 as the old-age threshold leads to the conclusion that an increasing proportion of adult lifetimes were being spent in old age.

When we compare Tables 6.1a and 6.1b, we see that the proportion of adult person-years spent in old age was 18 percent for Danes born in 1860, using age 65 as the old-age threshold, and 22 percent using the POAT. The proportion is higher when the POAT was used because for Danes born in 1860 remaining life expectancy fell to 15 years before they were 65 years old. For people born in 1920, the corresponding figures are higher when that proportion is assessed using age 65 as the old-age threshold and lower when it is assessed using the POAT.

Table 6.1a Proportions of adult person-years spent at age 65 or above, cohort life tables

Country	Year of birth			
	1860	1880	1900	1920
Denmark	0.18	0.20	0.22	0.24
England and Wales	0.16	0.19	0.21	0.23
Finland		0.16	0.19	0.24
France	0.15	0.18	0.21	0.26
Iceland	0.19	0.21	0.24	0.26
Italy		0.19	0.22	0.25
Netherlands	0.17	0.20	0.23	0.25
Sweden	0.18	0.20	0.23	0.26
Switzerland		0.18	0.22	0.26

Data sources: University of California, Berkeley, and Max Planck Institute for Demographic Research (2017); authors' calculations.

Note: Computed as T_{65}/T_{20} for each cohort and country, where T_x is the number of person-years lived from age x and onward. Data are for both sexes combined.

Table 6.1b Proportions of adult person-years spent at the prospective old-age threshold or above, cohort life tables

Country	Year of birth			
	1860	1880	1900	1920
Denmark	0.22	0.21	0.21	0.20
England and Wales	0.22	0.21	0.21	0.20
Finland		0.22	0.21	0.19
France	0.22	0.20	0.20	0.19
Iceland	0.20	0.20	0.20	0.20
Italy		0.21	0.21	0.19
Netherlands	0.22	0.21	0.21	0.20
Sweden	0.22	0.21	0.21	0.20
Switzerland		0.21	0.20	0.19

Data sources: University of California, Berkeley, and Max Planck Institute for Demographic Research (2017); authors' calculations.

Note: Computed as T_{POAT}/T_{20} for each cohort and country, where T_x is the number of person-years lived from age x and onward and $POAT$ is the prospective old-age threshold. Data are for both sexes combined.

Tables 6.1a and 6.1b are based on the same historical data, but what we see from the same data depends crucially on how we conceptualize age. If age 65 is used as the old-age threshold, we would observe increases in the percentage of adult lifetimes spent in old age between people born in 1860 and those born in 1920. If the POAT is used, we generally observe decreases in that percentage over the same period. If this trend continued, what proportions of adult person-years would be spent in old age in the future? There are no cohort life tables in the HMD that go much beyond the cohort born in 1920, but we can move toward answering this question using period life tables in the HMD.

Proportion of Adult Lifetime in Old Age Based on Period Life Tables from 1920–2010

With period life tables, we can compute the percentage of adult person-years lived in old age using the survival rates of a given year. In Table 6.2a, we show the proportions of adult person-years, those spent at age 20 and above, that are also spent at age 65 or above for the same nine countries as in Tables 6.1a and 6.1b, at 20-year intervals from 1920 through 2000 and for 2010.

Table 6.2a Proportions of adult person-years lived at age 65 or above, period life tables

Country	1920	1940	1960	1980	2000	2010
Denmark	0.18	0.18	0.21	0.23	0.25	0.27
England and Wales	0.17	0.16	0.20	0.22	0.26	0.28
Finland	0.15	0.13	0.18	0.22	0.26	0.28
France	0.16	0.14	0.21	0.24	0.28	0.30
Iceland	0.18	0.21	0.23	0.25	0.28	0.29
Italy	0.15	0.17	0.21	0.23	0.28	0.30
Netherlands	0.17	0.18	0.22	0.24	0.26	0.28
Sweden	0.19	0.19	0.22	0.24	0.27	0.29
Switzerland	0.14	0.17	0.21	0.24	0.28	0.30

Data sources: University of California, Berkeley, and Max Planck Institute for Demographic Research (2017); authors' calculations.

Note: Computed as T_{65}/T_{20} for each year and country, where T_x is the number of person-years lived from age x and onward. Data are for both sexes combined.

Table 6.2b Proportions of adult person-years spent at the prospective old-age threshold or above, period life tables

	1920	1940	1960	1980	2000	2010
Denmark	0.23	0.23	0.23	0.21	0.21	0.21
England and Wales	0.22	0.23	0.23	0.22	0.21	0.20
Finland	0.22	0.22	0.23	0.22	0.21	0.20
France	0.23	0.23	0.22	0.21	0.20	0.19
Iceland	0.22	0.22	0.21	0.21	0.20	0.21
Italy	0.23	0.24	0.22	0.22	0.21	0.20
Netherlands	0.23	0.23	0.22	0.21	0.21	0.20
Sweden	0.22	0.23	0.23	0.21	0.21	0.20
Switzerland	0.24	0.24	0.23	0.21	0.20	0.20

Data sources: University of California, Berkeley, and Max Planck Institute for Demographic Research (2017); authors' calculations.

Note: Computed as T_{POAT}/T_{20} for each year and country, where T_x is the number of person-years lived from age x and onward and $POAT$ is the prospective old-age threshold. Data are for both sexes combined.

In England and Wales, for example, the percentage of adult person-years spent at age 65 and above increases from 17 percent in 1920 to 28 percent in 2010. The findings for England and Wales are not an exception. In all the countries in Table 6.2a, the percentage of adult person-years spent at age 65 and above increases substantially.

In Table 6.2b, we show the analogous table using, instead, the POAT. The percentages of adult person-years spent in old age are roughly stable from 1920 to 1960 and then they fell slowly. Just as in Table 6.1a and 6.1b, Table 6.2a and 6.2b show that things look very different depending on which glasses we are wearing. Using the fixed chronological age of 65 as the old-age threshold, the proportion of the adult lifetime spent in old age increases over time; using the POAT that proportion decreases very slowly.

Proportion of Adult Lifetime in Old Age in the Future

We do not know what the future has in store for us, but we can use forecasted period life tables to see what the United Nations (2017e) expects to happen. In Table 6.3a, we present forecasts of the proportions of adult person-years spent in old age in Denmark, Finland, France,

Table 6.3a   Proportions of adult person-years lived at age 65 or above

	2015–2020	2045–2050	2095–2100
Denmark	0.32	0.34	0.38
Finland	0.33	0.35	0.39
France	0.34	0.37	0.40
Iceland	0.33	0.35	0.39
Italy	0.33	0.36	0.39
Netherlands	0.32	0.35	0.38
Sweden	0.33	0.35	0.39
Switzerland	0.33	0.36	0.39
United Kingdom	0.33	0.35	0.39

Data sources: United Nations (2017e); authors' calculations.
Note: Computed as T_{65}/T_{20} for each year and country, where T_x is the number of person-years lived from age x and onward for the year and country. Data are for both sexes combined.

Table 6.3b   Proportions of adult person-years lived at the prospective old-age threshold or above, period life tables

	2015–2020	2045–2050	2095–2100
Denmark	0.24	0.23	0.21
Finland	0.24	0.23	0.21
France	0.24	0.22	0.21
Iceland	0.24	0.22	0.21
Italy	0.24	0.22	0.20
Netherlands	0.24	0.23	0.21
Sweden	0.24	0.22	0.21
Switzerland	0.23	0.22	0.20
United Kingdom	0.24	0.23	0.21

Data sources: United Nations (2017e); authors' calculations.
Note: Computed as T_{POAT}/T_{20} for each year and country, where T_x is the number of person-years lived from age x and onward and *POAT* is the prospective old-age threshold for the year and country. Data are for both sexes combined.

Iceland, Italy, the Netherlands, Sweden, Switzerland, and the United Kingdom using 65 as the old-age threshold. For the selected countries, the proportion of adult person-years rises from around 30 percent in 2015–2020 to around 38 percent in 2095–2100.

We do not realistically expect that around 38 percent of adult life-times of people in the selected countries will be spent in old age by the end of the century, but this is the logical outcome of insisting that old age always begins at 65. We have a different, multidimensional view. In Table 6.3b, the forecasted proportions of adult person-years lived in old age are given using the prospective old-age threshold. From that perspective, we see that the proportion of adult person-years lived in old age falls slowly over time. The stage of old age, viewed that way, is forecasted to take up a progressively smaller proportion of the adult lifetime. Which glasses we use, again, makes a substantial difference here. With the old pair of glasses, it looks like the stage of old age will take up an ever-larger share of the adult lifetime. With our new glasses and multidimensional vision, the stage of old age appears to be taking a smaller proportion of the adult lifetime as the century progresses.

Which glasses we wear also affects how we perceive the speed of change in the proportion of the adult lifetime spent in old age. The use of age 65 as the old-age threshold produces what looks like relatively fast changes, while the use of the POAT shows slower changes. For example, the proportion for Sweden in Tables 6.3a and 6.3b increases from 0.35 to 0.39 from 2045–2050 to 2095–2100 when age 65 is used and decreases from 0.22 to 0.20 over the same period when the prospective threshold is used.

Health, as Reflected in 5-Year Death Rates, at the Onset of Old Age

Now that we know about the fraction of adult lifetimes spent in old age, let us move on to learn about people as they just enter the life cycle phase that we label as old age. Imagine that we stood at the gateway to old age, gave everyone who passed through it an identification number, and later used that number to determine the fraction of people who passed into old age and then died within 5 years. That 5-year death rate is closely correlated with the health of the people who enter old age. In our imaginary scenario, there are no wars, famines, or epidemics, so the 5-year death rate is one indicator of the health of those entrants. Health is, of course, itself a complex multidimensional phenomenon; 5-year death rates reflect only one of its many facets.

Table 6.4 presents the 5-year death rates of those who first cross the threshold into old age using cohort life tables from the HMD. What

Table 6.4   5-year death rates at two old-age thresholds, cohort life tables

	1860	1880	1900	1920
Denmark				
POAT	0.12	0.12	0.14	0.14
65	0.16	0.13	0.13	0.12
England and Wales				
POAT	0.13	0.13	0.14	0.14
65	0.19	0.15	0.15	0.12
Finland				
POAT		0.14	0.14	0.14
65		0.19	0.16	0.11
France				
POAT	0.13	0.14	0.14	0.12
65	0.19	0.15	0.13	0.09
Iceland				
POAT	0.13	0.12	0.14	0.13
65	0.14	0.12	0.11	0.08
Italy				
POAT		0.13	0.13	0.13
65		0.14	0.13	0.10
Netherlands				
POAT	0.12	0.13	0.13	0.13
65	0.17	0.13	0.12	0.10
Sweden				
POAT	0.12	0.13	0.13	0.12
65	0.15	0.13	0.11	0.09
Switzerland				
POAT		0.14	0.14	0.13
65		0.16	0.13	0.09

Data sources: University of California, Berkeley, and Max Planck Institute for Demographic Research (2017); authors' calculations.

Note: The 5-year death rates are proportions of people who die within 5 years of the old-age threshold assumed to be either age 65 or the prospective old-age threshold (POAT).

we see is that people born in 1860 and people born in 1920 had about the same death rate at their prospective old-age thresholds. For example, the 5-year death rate for people at the POAT was around 0.12 for people born 1860 and 0.13 for those born in 1880, 1900, and 1920. In contrast, the 5-year death rate generally fell when old age was assumed always to begin at age 65. People at the POAT who were born in 1860, 1880, 1900, and 1920 were about as healthy as one another in the dimension of

Table 6.5   5-year death rates at two old-age thresholds, period life tables

	1920	1940	1960	1980	2000	2010
Denmark						
POAT	0.12	0.12	0.11	0.13	0.13	0.11
65	0.16	0.16	0.12	0.12	0.10	0.07
England and Wales						
POAT	0.14	0.13	0.13	0.13	0.12	0.11
65	0.18	0.19	0.14	0.13	0.08	0.06
Finland						
POAT	0.14	0.14	0.12	0.12	0.11	0.10
65	0.20	0.22	0.16	0.12	0.08	0.06
France						
POAT	0.13	0.13	0.12	0.12	0.11	0.10
65	0.19	0.22	0.13	0.10	0.07	0.06
Iceland						
POAT	0.12	0.12	0.10	0.12	0.11	0.10
65	0.15	0.13	0.09	0.09	0.07	0.05
Italy						
POAT	0.13	0.12	0.12	0.12	0.11	0.10
65	0.19	0.17	0.13	0.11	0.07	0.05
Netherlands						
POAT	0.13	0.12	0.11	0.12	0.11	0.11
65	0.18	0.16	0.11	0.10	0.08	0.06
Sweden						
POAT	0.12	0.12	0.11	0.12	0.11	0.10
65	0.15	0.15	0.12	0.10	0.07	0.06
Switzerland						
POAT	0.13	0.12	0.12	0.12	0.10	0.10
65	0.23	0.18	0.13	0.10	0.07	0.05

Data sources: University of California, Berkeley, and Max Planck Institute for Demographic Research (2017); authors' calculations.

Note: The 5-year death rates are proportions of people who die within 5 years of the old-age threshold assumed to be either age 65 or the prospective old-age threshold (POAT).

health reflected in 5-year death rates. If we use age 65 as the old-age threshold, we see that people entering old age were much healthier in that dimension in 1920 than in 1860.

Table 6.5 provides the 5-year death rates using the two old-age thresholds, age 65 and the POAT, for the same countries and time periods as in Tables 6.2a and 6.2b. As in those tables, we use period life tables from the HMD. If age 65 is used as the old-age threshold, then

19 percent of the Italian entrants into old age would die within 5 years of entering in 1920. By 2010, only 5 percent would die within 5 years of their entrance into old age. The Italian experience is fairly typical of the countries in the table. When age 65 is used as the old-age threshold, the people who were entering old age in 2010 were far different from those who entered in 1920. The later entrants, having substantially lower 5-year death rates, appear to be far healthier in that dimension of health. If instead the POAT is used, health at the onset of old age declines more slowly. For example, between 1980 and 2010, the 5-year survival rate at the threshold of old age in Italy either falls by more than half, from 0.11 to 0.05 using the conventional old-age threshold, or falls more slowly from 0.12 to 0.10 using the prospective one. People at the POAT were more similar to one another over time and space in terms of 5-year survival rates than people at age 65.

Using forecasts from the United Nations, we show in Table 6.6 that we see the same pattern. In Italy, the 5-year death rate at the onset of old age either falls from 0.05 in 2015–2020 to 0.01 in 2095–2100 using age 65 as the old-age threshold, or from 0.10 to 0.07 over the same period using the POAT. Regardless of which old-age threshold is used, people at the onset of old age appear to be getting healthier over time, but people at the POAT in the future are likely to be more similar to people today at the POAT than 65-year-olds in the future are likely to be like today's 65-year-olds.

Conclusion

In this chapter, we learned that our view of whether people are spending a longer proportion of their adult lifetimes in old age depends on which glasses we are wearing. When we wear the old one-dimensional glasses, it looks like a greater and greater proportion of adult lifetimes is spent in old age. When we wear our multidimensional glasses, things look different. Over time, people will generally be spending lower proportions of their adult lifetimes in old age as time progresses.

Using the data in the tables in this chapter, we cannot answer the question about whether health in the life cycle stage of old age has been generally deteriorating or improving over time. We will address this question in Chapter 7. Here, we explored a simpler question, whether

Table 6.6 Forecasted 5-year death rates at two old-age thresholds,
period life tables

	2015–2020	2045–2050	2095–2100
Denmark			
POAT	0.11	0.10	0.08
65	0.06	0.04	0.02
Finland			
POAT	0.10	0.09	0.07
65	0.05	0.03	0.01
France			
POAT	0.10	0.08	0.07
65	0.05	0.03	0.01
Iceland			
POAT	0.10	0.09	0.06
65	0.05	0.03	0.01
Italy			
POAT	0.10	0.09	0.07
65	0.05	0.03	0.01
Netherlands			
POAT	0.10	0.09	0.07
65	0.05	0.03	0.01
Sweden			
POAT	0.10	0.08	0.06
65	0.05	0.03	0.01
Switzerland			
POAT	0.09	0.07	0.05
65	0.04	0.03	0.01
United Kingdom			
POAT	0.11	0.09	0.07
65	0.06	0.03	0.01

Data sources: United Nations (2017e); authors' calculations.

Note: The 5-year death rates are proportions of people who die within 5 years of
the old-age threshold assumed to be either age 65 or the prospective old-age
threshold (POAT).

the 5-year survival rates of people first entering the stage of old age has
changed over time. With both pairs of glasses, we saw that the 5-year
survival rates of people entering the stage of old age had been improving
and is forecasted to continue to improve in the future.

Using the prospective old-age threshold does not eliminate the
stage of old age. It measures its features differently. What we see is
the stage of old age encompassing a rather stable fraction of the adult

lifetime. Over time, 5-year death rates were decreasing slowly for people entering old age. What we do not see is also important. We do not see, with either pair of glasses, an ever-lengthening period of old age accompanied by higher 5-year death rates at its onset. If we think that age 65 is the appropriate old-age threshold for all countries and time periods, then the phase of old age did increase over time and the 5-year death rates of those entering old age improved as well.

There is a concern that, as life expectancy increases, people will be spending more time in poor health. To address this concern, it is necessary to formulate specific questions and to provide answers to them. Our first question was whether people will be spending an even greater proportion of their lives in the stage of old age. When we look at the stage of old age using the old glasses, we see that people will be spending increasing fractions of their adult lifetimes in the state of old age, but this is not what we see with the new glasses. Wearing the new glasses, we see that the stage of old age is forecasted to be a slowly decreasing portion of adult lifetimes. Wearing the old glasses, we see that 5-year death rates decrease at the onset of old age. We also see a decrease wearing the new glasses, albeit a slower one. In this chapter, we investigated one aspect of health in old age, the one reflected in 5-year death rates. With our multidimensional vision, we can see more dimensions of health in old age, so let's move on to explore them in Chapter 7.

7

Is the Quality of Life in Old Age Getting Worse?

IN CHAPTER 6, we explored the stage of old age. Using the 5-year survival rate as a rough indicator of health, we saw that health at the *prospective old-age threshold (POAT)* changed very little over time, even as the stage of old age began at progressively older chronological ages. In this chapter, we visit Europe to delve more deeply into the question of what has been happening to the health of people while in the stage of old age. We want to see whether old age in Europe has increasingly been spent in poor health.

In approaching this question, we use life tables augmented with data from surveys. Although life tables were developed for the study of patterns of mortality, they are now used in areas where it makes sense to think about people's characteristics in terms of categories, or what are more technically called "states." There are working life expectancy tables used to compute the expected number of years people are in the labor force. There are marital status life tables used to compute the number of years people are expected to be married, single, widowed, or divorced. There are life tables of people in various states of health. In this chapter, we investigate what we can see using life tables augmented with information about people's health and activity limitations.

Health-Related Life Tables

Remaining life expectancy at any specific age is the average number of years that people of that age are expected to live given the survival rates in the life table. Let us imagine that, in addition to the survival rates of people at each age, we also knew whether those people had some particular characteristic such as ill health, the ability to walk a mile without difficulty, or the ability to remember one's birthday. With age-specific data on the prevalence of the characteristic, it is possible to compute a characteristic-specific life expectancy—the number of years people of a given age would be expected to live while having the characteristic—using both the survival rates in the life table and the age-specific proportions of people who have the characteristic.

The technique of merging information about people's characteristics with life tables is called the Sullivan method (Sullivan 1971). The Sullivan method generally combines data from life tables, derived from censuses or registers and vital statistics, and information about people's characteristics derived from surveys.

The European Health and Life Expectancy Information System (EHLEIS, n.d.a) produced health-related life tables using data from 4 sets of surveys: the European Community Household Panel (ECHP), the European Social Survey (ESS), the Survey of Health, Ageing, and Retirement in Europe (SHARE), and the EU Statistics on Income and Living Conditions (EU-SILC). We use data from SHARE here because of its compatibility with other surveys.

SHARE is a sister survey to the Health and Retirement Study (HRS) in the United States (HRS, n.d.). HRS is a comprehensive survey of people who are 50 years old or older covering an astonishingly broad range of topics with well-tested and insightful questions. The success of the HRS has generated a set of sister surveys with largely identical questions. These sister surveys include, among others, the Canadian Longitudinal Study of Aging (CLSA), the Chinese Health and Retirement Longitudinal Study (CHARLS), the Costa Rican Longevity and Healthy Aging Study (CRELES), the English Longitudinal Study of Aging (ELSA), the Indonesian Family Life Survey (IFLS), the Irish Longitudinal Study of Ageing (TILDA), the Japanese Study of Aging and Retirement (JSTAR), the Korean Longitudinal Study of Ageing (KLoSA), the Mexican Health and Aging Study (MHAS), and the aforementioned Survey of Health, Ageing, and Retirement in Europe (SHARE). These surveys provide a rich source of data on population aging and the methods that we present in this chapter can readily be applied using information contained in them.

Health-Related Life Tables Based on SHARE Data

To create health-related life tables from these surveys requires combining health data with life table data using the Sullivan method. EHLEIS has already produced 8 sets of health-related life tables using SHARE data, saving us the step of combining the data ourselves. In this chapter, we use 4 sets of health-related life tables, allowing us to study the interaction of health and aging from different perspectives.

One dimension is the extent of physical functional limitations in old age. In SHARE, respondents are asked about their physical functional limitations. They were shown a card that listed possible functional limitations and were asked whether they had difficulty with each of them "because of a health or physical problem." They were explicitly instructed to ignore any limitations that they expected to last less than 3 months. The possible physical limitations were,

> having problems (1) walking 100 meters (a bit more than 100 yards), (2) sitting for about 2 hours, (3) getting up from a chair after sitting for long periods, (4) climbing several flights of stairs without resting, (5) climbing one flight of stairs without resting, (6) stooping, kneeling or crouching, (7) reaching or extending one's arms above shoulder level, (8) pulling or pushing large objects like a living room chair, (9) lifting or carrying weights over 10 pounds / 5 kilos, like a heavy bag of groceries, and (10) picking up a small coin from a table. (EHLEIS, n.d.c)

Based on the answers to these questions, we used, as a characteristic, the proportion of the population having no physical functional limitations.

A second dimension of health and aging is mental health. In SHARE, respondents were asked about limitations (called instrumental activity limitations) that they had "because of physical, mental, emotional, or memory" problems. People who reported instrumental activity limitations were having a problem (1) using a map to figure out how to get around in a strange place, (2) preparing a hot meal, (3) shopping for groceries, (4) making phone calls, (5) taking medications,

(6) doing work around the house or garden, and (7) managing money, such as paying bills and keeping track of expenses (EHLEIS, n.d.b). Based on answers to these questions, we used, as a characteristic, the proportion of the population having no instrumental activity limitations.

There is clearly some overlap in these questions. A person could have difficulty both lifting a heavy bag of groceries and have difficulty shopping for groceries. For the most part, though, they reflect different aspects of aging. The expected number of years of life without any physical functional limitations and the expected number of years of life without any instrumental activity limitations provide us with focused tools with which to analyze the health and aging of older people.

The characteristics, having no physical functional limitation and having no instrumental activity limitations, are derived from questions about specific activity limitations. SHARE also provides us with a more general question known as the Global Activity Limitations Indicator (GALI). The GALI is a single question developed by Euro-REVES (REVES, n.d.) for comparison of countries in the European Union: "For the past six months at least, to what extent have you been limited because of a health problem in activities people usually do?" Three answers are allowed: not limited, limited but not severely, and severely limited. The characteristic that we used based on the GALI was the proportion of the population having no activity limitations.

The GALI provides different information from what is obtained from the two other activity limitation questions. Those questions are based on lists of specific activities. The GALI asks about limitations "in activities people usually do." However, people in different countries, in different occupations, and at different ages do different things. The effects of physical and cognitive limitations are different in different environments. A person with severe mobility limitations who could not leave her house would report that she had physical functional limitations and could also report herself as being severely limited in answer to the GALI question. If, on the other hand, the person had an appropriately designed car and other mobility aids, she might report herself limited, but not severely, or possibly not limited at all because, with those devices, she could now do more or less what other people her age did. Men and women could answer the GALI question differently, as could people with different cultural backgrounds.

The extent of activity limitations also depends in part on the healthcare system. In the United States, for example, in 2000, 137 per 100,000 people aged 55–64 had hip replacements. By 2010, that number had increased to 253 per 100,000. In 2000, 249 per 100,000 people over 75 years old had hip replacements. By 2010, that number had increased to 418 per 100,000 people. The increase in obesity in the United States increases activity limitations and the demand for hip replacements. Hip transplants reduce activity limitations not only for the obese but for many others as well. Thus, the information provided in answers to questions on activity limitations is context dependent (Wolford, Palso, and Bercovitz 2015). Nevertheless, the GALI has been extensively tested and found to be informative and useful in a wide variety of contexts.

Activity limitations reduce the quality of life. Another factor reducing the quality of life is poor health. Activity limitations and health are related but not equivalent. A person needing a hip replacement could otherwise be in excellent health. A person in poor health could, nevertheless, report herself as not having any activity limitations. The fourth set of life tables that we use are based on people's responses to questions on their self-perceived health. People were asked to rate their health in five categories: excellent, very good, good, fair, and poor. People in different countries have different reporting styles, so cross-country comparisons need to be treated with caution, but variations over time within countries could still be meaningful. The characteristic that we used based on self-perceived health was the proportion of the population being in excellent, very good, or good health.

At this writing, the life tables produced by EHLEIS using SHARE data are available for the years 2004, 2006, 2010, and 2012. Other projects may produce similar life tables for later waves of SHARE, but we do not see any such life tables yet. Survey data on activity limitations and self-rated health are very sensitive to the details of how they are elicited. The order of questions could matter as well as a host of other hard to control variables. The data on physical functional limitations, instrumental activity limitations, and the GALI were collected reasonably consistently. However, the data on self-perceived health are consistent only for the years 2006, 2010, and 2012.

Now, using the four characteristic-specific life tables we discussed, and the POAT presented in Chapter 3, we are able to provide quantitative answers about health and aging. As life expectancy increases, the POAT increases indicating that old age begins at later ages. Using the POAT, people spend an average of 15 years in the state of old age. We address the relationship between health and aging by looking at the number of those years that are spent in four different states: (1) having no physical functional limitation, (2) having no instrumental functional limitations, (3) having no activity limitations, and (4) being in excellent, very good, or good self-rated health.

Tables 7.1–7.5 present those characteristics based on the EHLEIS life tables. In total, there are life tables for 18 countries and for the years 2004, 2006, 2010, and 2012. SHARE in 2008 asked questions in a different format, which is why data for that year are not included here. Further, not all countries have data for all 4 years. The averages in the tables in this chapter are for the countries for which data were available in all the years.

Table 7.1 shows the POATs that we use in our analysis. Generally, they increase over time. For women, the unweighted average of the POATs increased by 1.2 years from 2004 to 2012 and the average for men increased by 1.8 years. Using the POAT, we can see that, over time the onset of old age occurred later and later. But was this a cause of the deterioration of the quality of life within the period of old age?

We address this question first by looking at the number of years of expected life with none of the 10 functional activity limitations listed above starting at the POAT. In a particular year, if a person had even a single functional activity limitation, such as having difficulty getting up from a chair after sitting for long periods or climbing several flights of stairs without resting, that year would not be counted as one without any functional activity limitations. We present the expected number of years of expected life with no functional activity limitations within the period of old age beginning with the POAT in Table 7.2. The numbers for individual countries vary a bit because of statistical issues. In order to assess what has been happening more generally, we take unweighted averages over the countries for which data are available for all 4 years and assess its trend over time.

Table 7.1 Prospective old-age thresholds

	Women					Men			
	2004	2006	2010	2012		2004	2006	2010	2012
Austria	71.3	71.9	72.8	72.8	Austria	67.5	68.1	69.0	69.3
Belgium	71.3	71.9	72.8	72.8	Belgium	67.0	67.7	68.6	68.7
Czech Republic		69.2	70.1	70.4	Czech Republic		64.7	65.7	66.0
Denmark	70.3	70.4	71.0	71.7	Denmark	66.3	66.7	67.7	68.4
Estonia			70.8	71.7	Estonia			63.9	64.7
France	73.6	74.3	75.2	75.1	France	68.7	69.5	70.4	70.7
Germany	71.2	71.7	72.2	72.5	Germany	67.4	68.1	69.0	69.5
Greece	71.0	71.4			Greece	68.0	68.4		
Hungary			69.2		Hungary			63.5	
Italy	72.6	72.9	73.5	73.5	Italy	68.1	68.6	69.4	69.6
Luxembourg				73.0	Luxembourg				69.9
Netherlands	71.2	71.5	72.5	72.5	Netherlands	66.7	67.4	68.6	69.0
Poland		69.9	70.9		Poland		64.2	65.1	
Portugal			72.1		Portugal			68.1	
Slovenia			72.3	72.4	Slovenia			67.6	67.9
Spain	72.5	73.2	74.3	74.1	Spain	68.1	68.8	69.9	70.0
Sweden	72.1	72.3	72.6	72.4	Sweden	68.3	68.6	69.3	69.4
Switzerland	73.0	73.5	73.9	73.8	Switzerland	69.2	69.6	70.2	70.6
Average	71.9	72.4	73.1	73.1	Average	67.7	68.3	69.2	69.5

Data sources: EHLEIS (n.d.a); authors' calculations.
Note: For consistency, life tables in source are used.

The POAT is computed as the age at which remaining life expectancy is 15 years. In Table 7.2, we can see that, for women, around 3.5 of those 15 years were spent with no functional activity limitations and, for men, around 6.7 years of those years were spent with no functional activity limitations. Men spend more of their old age than women without any functional activity limitations for two reasons. First, they enter the stage of old age at a younger age, and second, their age-specific functional activity limitation rates tend to be lower. The most important feature of Table 7.2 is that there is no time trend in life expectancy without any functional activity limitations at the increasing POAT. In Table 7.1, we show that the average POAT for women increased from 71.9 in 2004 to 73.1 in 2012. Table 7.2 shows that, starting at age 71.9 in 2004, women's average life expectancy without any functional activity limitations was 3.4 years and that starting at age 73.1 in 2012, women's average life expectancy without any functional activity limitations was 3.5 years. Even though the onset of old age happened later in 2012, life expectancy without any functional activity limitations in the period of old age did not change. We see the same result for men.

Table 7.2 gives us one answer to the question about whether old age was becoming an increasingly unhealthy period of one's life. In old age, people had the same life expectancy without any functional activity limitations in 2004 as in 2012, even though the onset of old age was later in 2012. So, when we look at old age beginning at the prospective threshold, it did not become an increasingly difficult period, at least in terms of functional activity limitations.

In order to investigate the mental aspect of aging, we look at life expectancy, at the POAT, without any of the seven potential instrumental activity limitations listed earlier. We show those life expectancies in Table 7.3. Again, we see no trend in the averages. In 2004, the average POAT for men was 67.7 and it increased to 69.5 by 2012. Starting at age 67.7 in 2004, those men had a life expectancy without any instrumental activity limitations of 11.5 years. Starting at age 69.5 in 2012, they had a life expectancy without any instrumental activity limitations of 11.8 years. Even though the onset of old age was later in 2012, life expectancy without any instrumental activity limitations at the POAT was greater in 2012 than it was in 2004. There is no clear trend in life expectancy without any instrumental activity limitation

Table 7.2 Expected number of years of life with no physical functional limitations following the prospective old-age threshold

	Women				Men			
	2004	2006	2010	2012	2004	2006	2010	2012
Austria	3.2	3.0	3.6	3.0	6.9	6.2	6.0	6.5
Belgium	3.2	3.7	3.5	2.7	7.6	6.7	6.8	7.1
Czech Republic		2.8	2.3	3.1		7.4	7.6	7.3
Denmark	4.7	5.4	4.8	5.4	7.7	8.5	8.0	8.0
Estonia			2.7	2.5			6.6	5.7
France	2.7	2.5	2.2	2.5	5.7	6.4	5.6	5.5
Germany	2.5	2.4	3.1	3.3	5.4	5.1	5.1	6.5
Greece	1.6	1.3			4.6	4.7		
Hungary			3.3				5.1	
Italy	3.2	1.9	0.4	1.2	5.2	4.9	5.4	4.7
Luxembourg				2.8				6.0
Netherlands	4.4	5.1	5.6	5.3	7.9	8.5	8.5	8.3
Poland		1.4	2.1			4.3	6.0	
Portugal			1.8				4.7	
Slovenia			2.9	3.0			5.2	5.9
Spain	2.5	2.7	2.1	1.8	5.5	5.5	5.7	5.7
Sweden	3.5	2.9	3.8	4.8	6.5	7.1	7.0	8.1
Switzerland	4.5	5.7	4.7	5.0	7.2	8.2	7.7	7.7
Average	3.4	3.5	3.4	3.5	6.6	6.7	6.6	6.8

Data sources: EHLEIS (n.d.a); authors' calculations.
Note: For consistency, life tables in source are used.

at the POAT for either gender. It follows that old age was not becoming an increasingly undesirable period, at least in terms of instrumental activity limitations.

In Tables 7.2 and 7.3, we looked at life expectancies at the POAT free from any functional activity limitations and free from any instrumental activity limitations. We found that the duration of time in old age free from those limitations was about the same in 2012 as it was in 2004. But people could have limitations in activities that are not listed in the original surveys. To investigate this, we use the GALI question. In Table 7.4, we provide the results based on those who reported that they had no limitations in the activities that people usually do.

Table 7.4 shows that there is also no trend in life expectancy without any activity limitations at the POAT. In 2004, for women, the average life expectancy without any activity limitation at the POAT was 5.5 years and, in 2012, it was 5.3 years. For men, the analogous numbers were 7.0 and 7.2 years, respectively. Therefore, when we assess the quality of life in old age based on the GALI question, we again see that it was much the same in 2012 as it was in 2004, even though the POAT was higher in 2012. The analysis of activity limitations from three perspectives provides a consistent result. When the onset of old age is defined using the POAT, the resulting period of old age was one in which life expectancy without activity limitations did not significantly change.

An alternative approach to assessing the quality of life in old age is through questions on self-rated health. To do this, we defined the characteristic as being the proportion of the population in excellent, very good, or good health. We call people who report themselves in these categories "healthy" and use healthy life expectancies at the old-age threshold based on them. We show the results in Table 7.5, where we see that a healthy life expectancy for both men and women was highest in 2004. Between 2006 and 2012, there were increases for both genders. However, the question on self-rated health was asked differently in 2004 from the way it was asked in subsequent waves of the survey, so the 2004 figures need to be taken with caution. Starting in 2006, we see healthy life expectancy at the old-age threshold increasing.

Table 7.3 Expected number of years of life with no instrumental functional limitations following the prospective old-age threshold

	Women					Men			
	2004	2006	2010	2012		2004	2006	2010	2012
Austria	8.6	7.9	8.7	8.2	Austria	11.6	11.4	11.3	11.3
Belgium	8.2	8.1	7.9	6.5	Belgium	11.5	11.2	12.1	12.1
Czech Republic		9.8	8.4	9.0	Czech Republic		12.5	13.0	11.6
Denmark	9.3	9.2	10.5	10.2	Denmark	11.2	12.0	11.9	11.7
Estonia			8.0	7.9	Estonia			11.3	10.8
France	7.5	6.2	7.7	7.8	France	10.5	11.0	11.4	11.9
Germany	9.5	8.7	8.6	9.2	Germany	11.2	11.3	12.0	11.8
Greece	7.1	6.3			Greece	10.6	10.8		
Hungary			7.2		Hungary			10.1	
Italy	8.1	6.7	6.9	8.1	Italy	11.6	10.4	12.6	11.6
Luxembourg				8.4	Luxembourg				10.8
Netherlands	9.6	9.3	9.8	8.6	Netherlands	11.6	11.0	11.6	12.1
Poland		6.5	7.1		Poland		9.7	10.8	
Portugal			7.6		Portugal			11.2	
Slovenia			8.2	9.3	Slovenia			10.9	11.7
Spain	6.6	8.1	6.4	5.8	Spain	10.7	10.8	11.5	10.2
Sweden	8.3	9.2	9.6	10.8	Sweden	11.6	12.1	11.8	12.5
Switzerland	11.6	11.1	10.3	11.1	Switzerland	13.3	12.3	12.0	12.3
Average	8.7	8.4	8.6	8.7	Average	11.5	11.3	11.8	11.8

Data sources: EHLEIS (n.d.a); authors' calculations.
Note: For consistency, life tables in source are used.

Table 7.4 Expected number of years of life without self-reported limitations due to a health problem lasting at least the past 6 months in activities people usually do (GALI) following the prospective old-age threshold

	Women					Men			
	2004	2006	2010	2012		2004	2006	2010	2012
Austria	4.8	4.7	4.6	4.4	Austria	6.6	5.6	6.2	7.4
Belgium	5.9	5.6	5.1	4.6	Belgium	8.4	7.6	6.9	7.8
Czech Republic		3.3	3.4	4.6	Czech Republic		6.0	6.3	6.8
Denmark	5.8	6.6	6.7	7.0	Denmark	6.1	8.1	7.7	8.0
Estonia			3.6	3.3	Estonia			5.1	5.3
France	5.7	4.8	3.7	5.6	France	6.5	6.7	5.9	5.0
Germany	3.3	3.7	3.7	4.6	Germany	5.0	5.0	5.0	6.1
Greece	5.0	6.0			Greece	7.9	8.5		
Hungary			4.8		Hungary			5.7	
Italy	4.3	3.4	3.3	2.8	Italy	7.3	6.1	8.4	7.0
Luxembourg				4.8	Luxembourg				7.4
Netherlands	6.5	5.8	5.9	5.7	Netherlands	8.2	6.4	7.2	8.2
Poland		2.4	3.1		Poland		4.3	4.7	
Portugal			4.1		Portugal			5.7	
Slovenia			6.1	5.5	Slovenia			6.9	6.4
Spain	5.3	4.4	5.3	4.6	Spain	7.5	7.0	7.8	6.3
Sweden	5.8	5.3	5.9	6.2	Sweden	6.7	7.1	6.7	7.8
Switzerland	7.7	7.5	7.3	7.9	Switzerland	7.9	7.8	8.4	8.4
Average	5.5	5.2	5.1	5.3	**Average**	7.0	6.7	7.0	7.2

Data sources: EHLEIS (n.d.a); authors' calculations.
Note: For consistency, life tables in source are used.

Table 7.5 Expected number of years of life with positively assessed health following the prospective old-age threshold

	Women					Men			
	2004	2006	2010	2012		2004	2006	2010	2012
Austria	8.0	7.1	7.4	7.9	Austria	9.3	9.6	8.9	9.4
Belgium	8.6	8.2	8.3	9.2	Belgium	9.9	9.5	10.5	10.6
Czech Republic		5.3	5.1	4.7	Czech Republic		7.8	8.8	8.2
Denmark	9.3	9.4	9.3	9.3	Denmark	10.1	10.6	9.8	10.4
Estonia			1.9	2.0	Estonia			3.3	3.1
France	7.0	5.0	5.9	6.5	France	7.1	6.7	7.3	7.1
Germany	5.5	5.4	6.3	6.6	Germany	7.1	6.3	6.7	7.3
Greece	6.0	6.9			Greece	8.4	9.0		
Hungary			4.6		Hungary			5.5	
Italy	4.8	3.8	1.9	5.8	Italy	7.2	6.1	7.6	6.6
Luxembourg				7.7	Luxembourg				8.9
Netherlands	8.8	8.6	8.8	7.7	Netherlands	9.7	8.7	9.0	9.0
Poland		2.5	2.3		Poland		3.7	4.8	
Portugal			0.7		Portugal			5.3	
Slovenia			6.2	7.0	Slovenia			6.4	7.8
Spain	5.4	4.1	5.2	4.5	Spain	8.3	6.2	7.3	6.6
Sweden	11.9	7.4	7.3	8.3	Sweden	12.3	9.7	9.4	10.2
Switzerland	11.6	11.3	10.1	10.4	Switzerland	11.4	10.8	10.3	11.3
Average	8.1	7.0	7.1	7.6	Average	9.2	8.4	8.7	8.9

Data sources: EHLEIS (n.d.a); authors' calculations.
Note: For consistency, life tables in source are used.

Conclusion

Given the survival rates in a life table, people at the POAT would live an average of 15 more years. When we observe the life expectancy of people at the POAT without activity limitations, we are seeing what fraction of those remaining years are spent without any activity limitations. Consider two populations, for example, population 1 observed in 2006 and population 2 observed in 2012. Let the POAT in population 1 be 70 and the POAT in population 2 be 72. If life expectancy without any activity limitations were 5 years in both, it means that 70-year-old people in population 1 would have an average of 15 more years of life and that those people would also have an average of 5 more years of life without any activity limitations. It also means that 72-year-old people in population 2 would have an average of 15 more years of life and that those people, too, would have an average of 5 more years of life without any activity limitations. In this example, the onset of old age is later in population 2 than in population 1, but the quality of life in old age, as measured by the prevalence of activity limitations, is the same in both populations. This is essentially what we observe here. The evidence that we have presented above is not consistent with the idea that the period of old age has been becoming one of decreasing quality of life, at least with the measures that we have been able to use. If anything, there is tentative evidence of the reverse. A conservative conclusion is that the quality of life in old age in the populations we studied has not diminished over time even as the POAT has increased.

This conclusion, however, must be considered tentative for several reasons. It is based on a subset of European countries over a period of 8 years. The results could be different if different countries or time periods are used. They could also be different if different criteria of the quality of life are used. Variations across time for individual countries can have an element of randomness because of statistical reasons. Responses to questions on activity limitations and health can vary with culture. They can also vary by age and gender because of a country's policies. People near the minimum age for a disability pension might be more likely to report themselves limited and in poor health. Therefore, caution must be exercised before concluding that people in one country are less limited or healthier than people in another or that people of a certain age appear to be unusually unhealthy. Also, many surveys, such as SHARE, are not designed to focus on health topics. Statistical details such as sample sizes, the nature of population heterogeneity, the replacement of people who leave the sample, and the geographic clustering of initial respondents and their replacements often cannot be fully addressed, resulting in less precise estimates than we would like. We deal with this lack of precision by taking averages. This helps us see general patterns, but single observations on countries and years need to be treated with caution.

Keeping these caveats in mind, what is important here is not what we see but what we do not see. In the countries for which we have data, we do not see the period of old age becoming a less healthy one.

This paper uses data from SHARE Waves 1, 2, 3 (SHARELIFE), 4, 5, and 6 (DOIs: 10.6103 / SHARE.w1.600, 10.6103 / SHARE.w2.600, 10.6103 / SHARE.w3.600, 10.6103 / SHARE.w4.600, 10.6103 / SHARE.w5.600, 10.6103 / SHARE.w6.600); see Börsch-Supan et al. (2013) for methodological details.

The SHARE data collection has been primarily funded by the European Commission through FP5 (QLK6-CT-2001-00360), FP6 (SHARE-I3: RII-CT-2006-062193, COMPARE: CIT5-CT-2005-028857, SHARELIFE: CIT4-CT-2006-028812), and FP7 (SHARE-PREP: N°211909, SHARE-LEAP: N°227822, SHARE M4: N°261982).

Additional funding from the German Ministry of Education and Research, the Max Planck Society for the Advancement of Science, the US National Institute on Aging (U01_AG09740-13S2, P01_AG005842, P01_AG08291, P30_AG12815, R21_AG025169, Y1-AG-4553-01, IAG_BSR06-11, OGHA_04-064, HHSN271201300071C), and various national funding sources is gratefully acknowledged (see www.share-project.org).

8

Survival Trajectories: Russian Regions and US States

IN CHAPTER 7, we found that our new glasses were helpful in seeing how health in old age has evolved in several European countries. In this chapter, we travel both to the east and to the west of those countries and investigate patterns of aging in the Russian Federation and the United States. Imagine, for a moment, that we would want to do this with our old glasses on. We would not be able to distinguish a 65-year-old Russian in Moscow from a 65-year-old Russian in Tuva or a 65-year-old American in Massachusetts from one in Mississippi. Fortunately, there is a way to improve our vision and make our trip more interesting, but it requires wearing the new glasses. We prepare for our journey by introducing a new way of visualizing, conceptualizing, and quantifying population aging in subgroups of populations such as people living within different regions of a country. Then we travel around the Russian Federation and the United States and see new dimensions of population aging there that were previously invisible.

Age Difference Trajectories

In Chapter 5, we introduced the concept of *α-ages*. These are ages based on characteristics of people. α-ages are always comparative. They tell us the age in a *standard population* where people have the same level of a specific characteristic as people of a given age in the population that we are considering. Consider, for example, looking at people who were 60 years old in a particular Russian region or US state who had a characteristic level of 10. To obtain their α-age, we would go to the relevant standard population to determine the age where people in that population had a characteristic level of 10. One possibility is that people in the standard population had a characteristic level of 10 at age 65. If the characteristic were remaining life expectancy, then people in the standard population get to live 5 years longer than the people in the region or state we are considering before their remaining life expectancy fell to the same level. If people in that region or state had an α-age of 65 when their chronological age was 60, it means that they had aged more rapidly than people in the standard population. Roughly speaking, when people's α-ages are higher than their chronological ages, they are older than their chronological ages indicate, when assessed relative to people in the standard population. When people's α-ages are lower than their chronological ages they are younger, in terms of the characteristic used, than their chronological ages indicate.

Whenever we compute α-ages we get a new measure as a bonus: the differences between α-ages and chronological ages. In the example above, the difference was 5 years; so, people's characteristic age, so to speak, was 5 years older than their chronological age, given the standard population that was used. We call the differences between α-ages and chronological ages *age differences*. In the old, one-dimensional world, no such differences exist.

Age Differences: Examples

We use *age difference trajectories* in this chapter as the basis of a new way of looking at population aging, one constructed by arraying age differences by chronological age. We present a hypothetical example of one in Table 8.1, using three chronological ages 45, 60, and 75.

In Table 8.1, the α-ages of people in population 1 are always 5 years higher than their chronological ages. In population 1, in terms of chronological ages, people 75 years old are 30 years older than those who are 45 years old. In terms of their α-ages, they are also 30 years older. The 75-year-olds had an α-age of 80 and the 45-year-olds had an α-age of 50. People in population 1 are older than people in the standard population

Table 8.1 Hypothetical example of two populations with constant
age differences

	Chronological age (standard population)		
	45	60	75
Population 1			
α-age	50	65	80
Age difference	5	5	5
Population 2			
α-age	40	55	70
Age difference	−5	−5	−5

Note: The α-ages are assumed to be computed based on the same characteristic.
The same standard population is assumed to be used in the computation of the
α-ages of the two populations.

given the characteristic that we are using in the comparison, but
people in the two populations were aging at the same pace.

Table 8.1 allows us to separate two important aspects of aging: differences in levels and differences in trends. People in population 1 are
older than people in the standard population at each age. They were
already older at age 45, but after age 45 the pace of aging is the same in
both populations; the age difference is constant at 5 years. After age
45, people in population 1 were not growing older faster than people in
the standard population.

In Table 8.1, people in population 2 are younger than people in the
standard population; the age difference is −5 years at each of the ages.
Nevertheless, they age at the same rate as people in the standard population since the difference between the chronological ages of
75-year-olds and 45-year-olds is 30 years and the difference between the
α-ages of 45- and 75-year-olds in population 2 is also 30 years.

Table 8.2 presents another pattern that we observe in age difference
trajectories. In Table 8.2, age differences increase with chronological
age. In population 1, over the 30 years from age 45 to age 75, α-ages increased by 34 years, from 46 to 80, and the age difference increased
from 1 year at age 45 to 5 years at age 75. An increasing age difference
indicates that the population is aging faster than the standard population. In Table 8.2, people in population 1 are older than people in the

Table 8.2   Hypothetical example of two populations with increasing
             age differences

	Chronological age (standard population)		
	45	60	75
Population 1			
α-age	46	63	80
Age difference	1	3	5
Population 2			
α-age	40	57	74
Age difference	−5	−3	−1

Note: The α-ages are assumed to be computed based on the same characteristic.
The same standard population is assumed to be used in the computation of the
α-ages of the two populations.

Table 8.3   Hypothetical example of two populations with decreasing
             age differences

	Chronological age (standard population)		
	45	60	75
Population 1			
α-age	50	63	76
Age difference	5	3	1
Population 2			
α-age	44	57	70
Age difference	−1	−3	−5

Note: The α-ages are assumed to be computed based on the same characteristic.
The same standard population is assumed to be used in the computation of the
α-ages of the two populations.

standard population, as indicated by their positive age differences and
they are aging faster as indicated by their increasing age differences.
People in population 2 are younger than people in the standard population as indicated by their negative age differences. They are also aging
faster as indicated by their increasing age differences.

   In Table 8.3, we present a third pattern sometimes seen in the data.
In this example, age differences are decreasing with chronological age.
Population 1 is again older than the standard population and population

2 is younger. Both populations are aging more slowly than the standard population. This is evident because, in both populations, people are 30 years older, chronologically, at 75 than they were at 45, but only 26 years older in terms of their α-ages.

In short, differences between α-ages and chronological ages and age difference trajectories provide a new way of looking at population aging. At a given chronological age, when the age difference is positive, it indicates that, at that age, the population is older than the standard population, in terms of the characteristic that is used. When the age difference is negative, the population is younger than the standard population. Changes in age differences over chronological age indicate how fast the population is aging relative to the standard population. When the age differences are constant, the population is aging at the same pace as the standard population. When age differences are increasing, the population is aging faster than the standard population and when those differences are decreasing, the population is aging more slowly.

Age Differences: An Example in the Literature

Milligan and Wise (2011) provide an interesting example of the use of age differences. For Sweden and the United States, they calculated what we would refer to as α-ages using 1-year mortality rates and proportions of population with poor self-assessed health as characteristics. They looked at people who were around age 60 in the mid-1970s and computed their α-ages using corresponding characteristic schedules about 3 decades later. What they found was that the age differences (differences between α-ages and chronological ages) were larger in both countries when self-assessed poor health was used than when 1-year mortality rates were used. In particular, age differences around age 60 in the mid-1970s, using self-assessed poor health as the characteristic, were approximately 9 years using a standard from around the mid-2000s, while the comparable age differences using mortality rates were around 7 to 8 years. These figures indicate that the improvement in the health measure was slightly faster than the improvement in mortality. This is consistent with what we saw when we looked at measures of health in Chapters 6 and 7.

Age Difference Trajectories in Russia and the United States

Now, let us continue our journey to the Russian Federation and the United States. The age differences and trajectories that we present here use 10-year survival rates as the characteristic. Recall, in the Chapter 5 appendix, we showed that the results in this chapter would be identical regardless of whether we used 10-year survival rates or 10-year death rates. This feature of age differences and age difference trajectories is crucial both here and for the wider applicability of these measures.

We use 10-year survival rates here for several reasons. First, their use provides an example of how characteristics other than remaining life expectancy can be used in studies of population aging. Second, we use 10-year survival rates instead of survival rates over shorter periods because they are less subject to random variability and express the underlying patterns of survival more clearly.

When we look at regional patterns in the Russian Federation and the United States, we are not discussing how Russia or the United States compare with the rest of the world, as both countries have unique demographic features. In Russia, male life expectancy is exceptionally low compared to female life expectancy. In the United States, life expectancy for both sexes is low compared to other countries with similar levels of per capita income. In this chapter, we look within countries and focus on regional differences that attract our attention. Sometimes, the differences reflect cultural differences between regions. Sometimes, they are noteworthy to us because they present puzzles that we have yet to understand.

Regional Age Difference Trajectories in the Russian Federation

The Russian Federation is vast, not only in the size of its territory, but also in the heterogeneity of its population. In 2000, the Russian Federation was divided into eight federal districts: five geographically smaller districts in the west and three larger ones in the east. The Central Federal District is the industrial heartland of the Russian Federation and includes Moscow. The Northwestern Federal District has two different parts. To the west, there is Saint Petersburg and its surrounding area, and, farther to the east, is the northernmost part of European Russia with its semi-Arctic climatic conditions. South of the Central Federal District in European Russia are two districts, the Southern Federal District, and, farther south, the Northern Caucasian Federal District. The Northern Caucasian Federal District is the southernmost district in European Russia and has a predominantly Muslim population. The Volga Federal District lies to the east of the Central District between the Northwestern Federal District and the Southern Federal District. Moving to the east from the five western districts are three districts that reach from the northernmost to the southernmost borders of the country. Moving from west to east, they are the Ural Federal District, the Siberian Federal District, and the Far-Eastern Federal District.

In this chapter, we compute age difference trajectories using data for Russian regions for 2015 (RANEPA, Rosstat, and IIASA 2016). As a standard, we use data in the Russian Federation as a whole in that year. In Table 8.4, we present age differences for Russian federal districts for men and women who were 55, 65, and 75 years old. Most of the age differences are positive. In those cases, populations had lower 10-year survival rates than the Russian Federation as a whole. The Central Federal District and the North Caucasian Federal District stand out because of their negative age differences. We also see negative age differences for men at all three ages and for women age 55 in the Southern Federal District.

In Table 8.4, two federal districts stood out as being significantly different from the rest—the Central Federal District and the North Caucasian Federal District—so we will hike over there to see what is going on. We will also travel to the Northwestern Federal District, home of Saint Petersburg, to have a look around there as well. On our journeys through the Russian Federation and the United States, we are aware that levels and trends in age difference trajectories are influenced by many factors, among them are behavioral differences and health system differences. The trajectories that we present will not allow us to say what factors cause their differences, but they can help us think about those issues from a firmer evidentiary base.

We first travel to Moscow. In Figure 8.1, we present the age difference trajectories for the city of Moscow and for Moscow Oblast, the area surrounding it. Figure 8.1a shows that 45-year-old women in Moscow had an

Table 8.4   Age differences for major Russian regions, 2015, men and
women, 55, 65, and 75 years old

District	Women			Men		
	55	65	75	55	65	75
Central Federal District	−1.26	−0.81	−0.34	−1.04	−1.38	−1.16
Northwestern Federal District	0.44	−0.44	−0.23	0.53	−0.40	−0.44
Southern Federal District	−0.68	0.03	0.26	−1.01	−0.77	−0.32
North Caucasian Federal District	−3.19	−1.19	−0.03	−4.47	−3.21	−2.09
Volga Federal District	−0.09	0.06	0.13	0.76	1.01	0.99
Ural Federal District	0.44	0.50	0.09	0.68	1.05	1.19
Siberian Federal District	2.06	0.98	0.19	1.36	1.43	1.19
Far-Eastern Federal District	2.73	2.02	0.91	2.56	2.81	1.56

Data sources: RANEPA, Rosstat, and IIASA (2016); authors' calculations.
Note: The standard population is the entire population of the Russian Federation.

age difference of −8.1 years from the national standard. This indicates
that their 10-year survival rate was the same as 36.9-year-old women in
the entire country. At older ages, the age differences converge to the Russian average, increasing to −3.4 years at age 60 and −2.4 years at age 75.

For men in Moscow, Figure 8.1a shows that differences from the
national average were greater than they were for women. At age 45, the
age difference was −11.2 years, indicating that 45-year-old men in
Moscow had the same 10-year survival rate as 33.8-year-olds in the entire Russian Federation. At age 60, the age difference is −6.7 years and
at age 75 it is −7.2 years. At all of the ages from 45 to 75, people in
Moscow have higher 10-year survival rates than people of those ages
in the country as a whole, and this is particularly true for men.

The large negative numbers for women and men in Moscow are due
in part to the relatively low survival rates of women and men in a
country with the Russian Federation's level of income and education.
In Moscow, however, those women and men have much higher survival rates, not unlike those of their counterparts in Western European
countries. That Moscow probably has the best healthcare in the Russian Federation may play a role here.

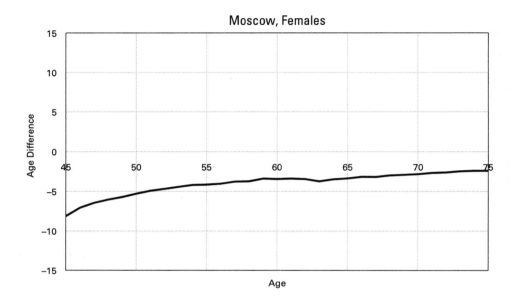

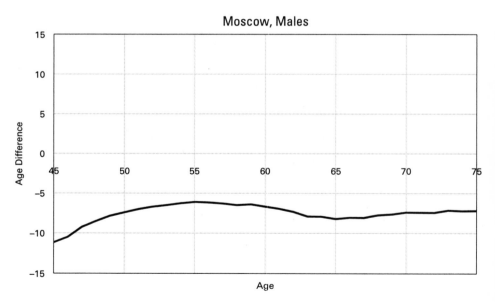

FIGURE 8.1A: Age difference trajectories for Moscow, women and men, 2015. Standard population is the population of the Russian Federation as a whole.

Data sources: RANEPA, Rosstat, and IIASA (2016); authors' calculations.

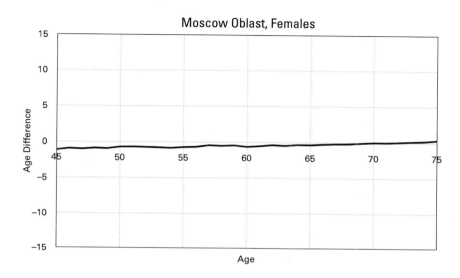

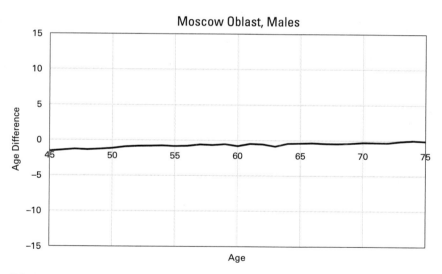

FIGURE 8.1B: Age difference trajectories for Moscow Oblast, women and men, 2015. Standard population is the population of the Russian Federation as a whole.

Data sources: RANEPA, Rosstat, and IIASA (2016); authors' calculations.

In Figure 8.1, we can also compare the age difference trajectories of people in Moscow to those of people in the Moscow Oblast. The age difference trajectories of people in Moscow Oblast differ markedly from those in the city of Moscow. The large negative age differences at age 45 are not seen there, nor are the marked differences by gender. In general, the age difference trajectory starts a bit below –1 at age 45 for both sexes and increases slowly toward 0. Aging in the Moscow Oblast is much more like in Russia as a whole than is the case for Moscow city.

The differences in patterns of aging in Moscow and Moscow Oblast are striking. The people in those two places are not especially different culturally, although that does not preclude consequential behavioral differences. Healthcare in Moscow is more advanced than in Moscow Oblast, but for advanced medical treatments people in Moscow Oblast would not need to travel far to get treatment in Moscow city.

Our next stop is Saint Petersburg. First, we visit the city and then its surrounding area, called Leningrad Oblast. We present the age difference trajectories for those areas in Figure 8.2. When we arrived in Saint Petersburg, we were struck by how different aging looked there compared to Moscow. The age difference trajectories of women in Saint Petersburg look quite different from those in Moscow. In Moscow, the age difference of 45-year-old women from the national standard was –8.1, while, in Saint Petersburg, it is –2.03. In Saint Petersburg, the age difference at age 75 is –1.51, only around half a year higher than at age 45. For women in Moscow, the difference between people at age 45 and 75 was much greater. Women in Saint Petersburg age much like women in the entire country, but women in Moscow do not.

The age difference trajectory for men in Saint Petersburg bears some similarities to the one observed in Moscow. In Moscow, after age 50, the age difference trajectory was roughly constant at –7.0. In Saint Petersburg, it is roughly constant at –3.5. After age 50, men in Saint Petersburg and Moscow aged at about the same pace as men in Russia as a whole, but men in Moscow had higher survival rates at each age.

Unexpectedly, the patterns of aging in Saint Petersburg seem more like those of Moscow Oblast than Moscow city. It is also interesting that the patterns of aging in Saint Petersburg and Leningrad Oblast are more like one another than those for Moscow and Moscow Oblast. In Leningrad Oblast, the age difference trajectory for women tends to be about 1.5 years higher than in Saint Petersburg, but, in both, there is not much change with age. For men, after age 50, both trajectories are roughly flat, with the one for Leningrad Oblast lying about 3.5 years higher. In a four-way comparison of Moscow city, Saint Petersburg, Moscow Oblast, and Leningrad Oblast, Moscow city stands out as being the most atypical.

Now we will travel southward to Russia's southernmost region, the Republic of Dagestan located in the North Caucasian region. Dagestan is a mountainous region. Its eastern border is the Caspian Sea. On its northern border is Stavropol Krai to which we will compare it. The comparison is of interest because while the Republic of Dagestan and Stavropol Krai are neighboring areas, the population of the Republic of Dagestan is a predominantly Muslim region while the population of Stavropol Krai is not. The Republic of Dagestan is one of the Russian Federation's most ethnically diverse regions.

As shown in Figure 8.3, 45-year-old Dagestani women had an age difference of −14.8, so they had the same 10-year survival rates as 30.2-year-olds in the Russian standard; while 45-year-old Dagestani men had an age difference of −15.6, so they had the same 10-year survival rate as 29.4-year-old men in Russia. In none of the other comparisons presented here do we see such large negative age differences. For both women and men, the differences approach 0 with increasing age, with the increase being much faster for women. The Republic of Dagestan is neither wealthy nor is it known for having especially good healthcare. Nevertheless, its age difference trajectories lie below those for Moscow city. Part of the explanation of this difference could well be differences in behavioral factors related to alcohol consumption, which is forbidden in the Quran.

Stavropol Krai lies just north of the Republic of Dagestan. Besides having a diversified economy, Stavropol Krai sports some of Russia's most famous health spas and recreational areas. The age difference for 45-year-old women in Stavropol Krai was −5.3 years, much higher than the −14.8 years observed for women in nearby Dagestan but still below the Russian average. For men in Stavropol Krai, the age difference at 45 was −3.0 years. For people of both genders, the age differences rise toward 0 with increasing age. The pattern of aging in Stavropol Krai is not that different from what we saw in Saint Petersburg.

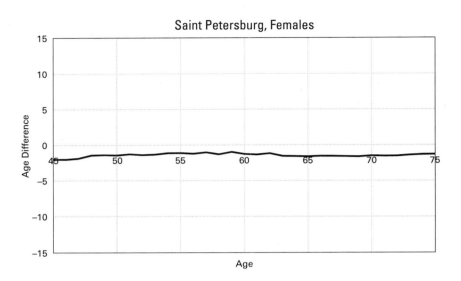

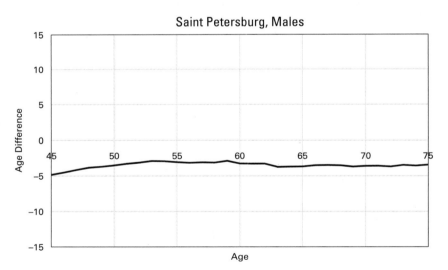

FIGURE 8.2A: Age difference trajectories for Saint Petersburg, women and men, 2015. Standard population is the population of the Russian Federation as a whole.

Data sources: RANEPA, Rosstat, and IIASA (2016); authors' calculations.

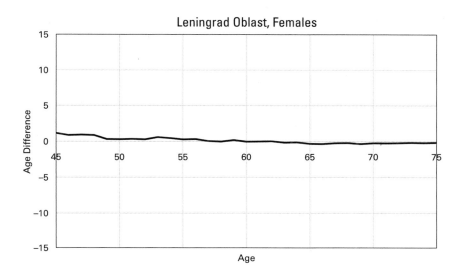

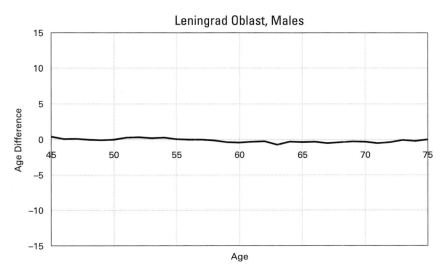

FIGURE 8.2B: Age difference trajectories for Leningrad Oblast, women and men, 2015. Standard population is the population of the Russian Federation as a whole.

Data sources: RANEPA, Rosstat, and IIASA (2016); authors' calculations.

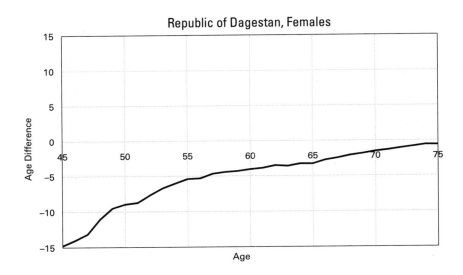

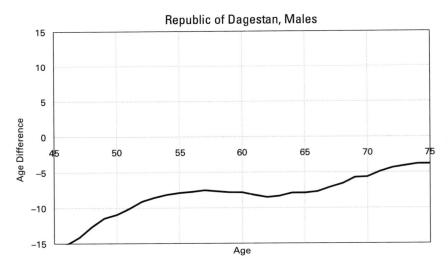

FIGURE 8.3A: Age difference trajectories for Republic of Dagestan, women and men, 2015. Standard population is the population of the Russian Federation as a whole.

Data sources: RANEPA, Rosstat, and IIASA (2016); authors' calculations.

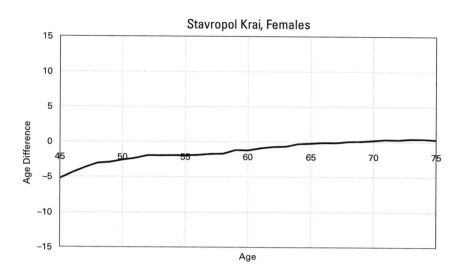

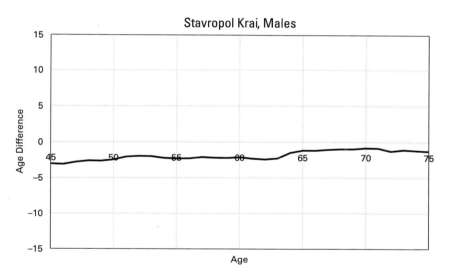

FIGURE 8.3B: Age difference trajectories for Stavropol Krai, women and men, 2015. Standard population is the population of the Russian Federation as a whole.

Data sources: RANEPA, Rosstat, and IIASA (2016); authors' calculations.

More information about aging in the Russian Federation can be found at RANEPA, Rosstat, and IIASA (2016) and Federal State Statistics Service, Russian Federation (n.d.).

Age Difference Trajectories in the United States

When we arrived in the United States, we found that life expectancy at birth there had barely changed during the first half of the 2010 decade. In fact, life expectancy at birth in 2010 (both sexes) was 78.7 years and it was also 78.7 years in 2015 (Xu et al. 2018, 26, table 4). For consistency, we analyze age difference trajectories for US states using data for 2015, the same year that we used for the Russian Federation. The data that we use come from the United States Mortality Database (University of California, Berkeley, n.d.), and we use women and men in the entire country as standard populations.

We began our trip to the Russian Federation by visiting the city of Moscow. Moscow is one of the regions of the Russian Federation with the highest survival rates for older people. To be comparable, we begin our trip to the United States in Washington, DC. We compared the age difference trajectory of Moscow with that of the surrounding Moscow Oblast. We cannot do that for Washington, DC, which is bounded on the north by the state of Maryland and on the south by the state of Virginia. We have chosen Maryland for comparison. It is more industrial than Virginia and, therefore, a bit more like Moscow Oblast. We show the comparison in Figure 8.4. In Moscow, age difference trajectories were negative throughout the age range indicating that survival rates there were much better than the national average. For men the age differences were large, usually being between −5 and −10 years. In Washington, DC, we see the opposite, very large positive age differences especially between ages 45 and 60. In those ages, survival rates were much worse than in the United States as a whole. The low survival rates of people between the ages of 45 and 60, skews the remaining population toward those who are more robust and the age difference trajectories converge toward the national average with increasing age.

The pattern of aging in Moscow Oblast differs markedly from that of Moscow. It looks very much like the pattern of aging in Russia as a whole. We see the same thing when we look at the age difference trajectory for Maryland. It looks like the trajectory of aging in the United States as a whole. In both countries, the capital cities have a distinctive pattern of aging that is very different from the national average while the areas adjacent to them do not.

After we visited Moscow and Moscow Oblast, we moved north and west to Saint Petersburg and Leningrad Oblast, so, from the mid-Atlantic region of the United States, we travel north and west to two states on the Canadian border, Michigan and Minnesota. An important difference between these states is their economic structures. Michigan is famed for being the heartland of America's automobile industry, but, as the industry there faced increasing difficulties, so did the parts of the state that relied on it. In one city, Flint, Michigan, the financial consequences of shuttered factories led, through a series of events, to the citizens of the city being exposed to high levels of lead in their drinking water. Minnesota, in contrast, has a much more diversified economy with substantial mining, agricultural, and financial sectors, as well as an industrial one. We show the comparison of their age difference trajectories in Figure 8.5.

The age difference trajectories for Michigan consistently lie somewhat above 0, showing that survival rates there are below the US average. In Minnesota, in contrast, the age difference trajectories are all negative from age 40 to age 85. In particular, relative survival rates are particularly high for people in the ages from 40 to 60. Between ages 40 and 50, the age difference trajectories are relatively flat in both states. At those ages, people in both places were aging at about the same rate as in the entire country, but the levels of survival rates were much higher in Minnesota.

Next, we travel westward to the states of Utah and Nevada, two states that border one another. Both are in the mountainous region in the western part of the country and both have areas of desert. Culturally, however, they are very different. Utah is the home of the Church of Jesus Christ of Latter-day Saints, often referred to as Mormon Church. The Mormon religion, like Islam, forbids the drinking of alcohol and encourages family solidarity. We look at Utah here because, in terms of attitudes toward alcohol consumption, it is the closest comparison in the United States to the Republic of Dagestan in the Russian Federation. Nevada is America's gambling capital and is home to the only legal brothels in the country. It is famous for its "what happens in Vegas stays in Vegas" attitude. Unlike Stavropol Krai, Nevada

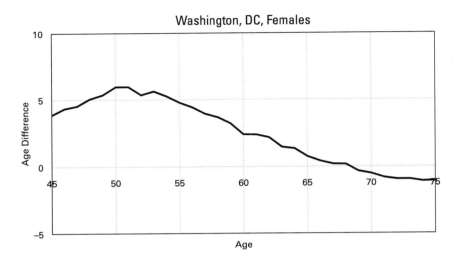

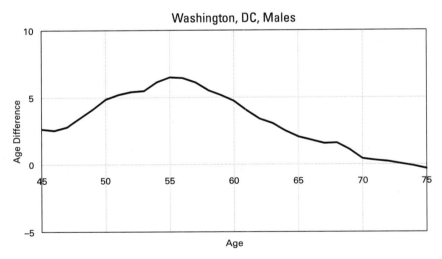

FIGURE 8.4A: Age difference trajectories for Washington, DC, women and men, 2015. Standard population is the population of the United States as a whole.

Data sources: University of California, Berkeley (n.d.); authors' calculations.

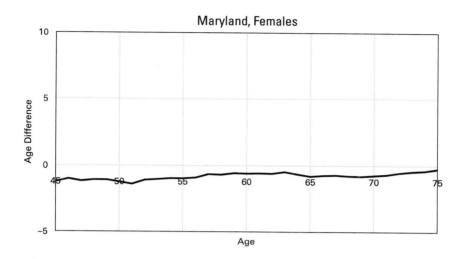

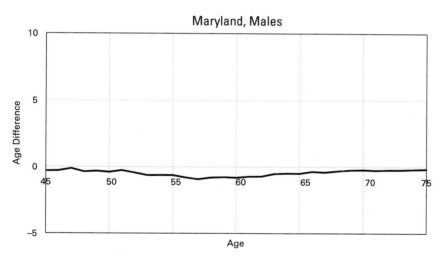

FIGURE 8.4B: Age difference trajectories for Maryland, women and men, 2015. Standard population is the population of the United States as a whole.

Data sources: University of California, Berkeley (n.d.); authors' calculations.

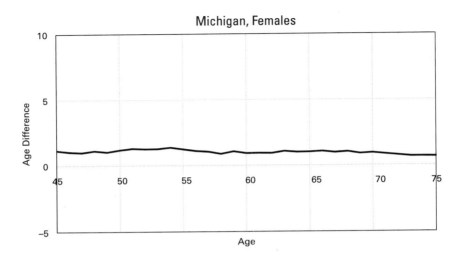

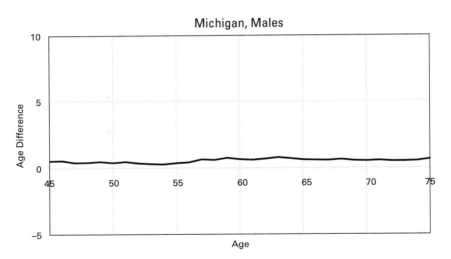

FIGURE 8.5A: Age difference trajectories for Michigan, women and men, 2015. Standard population is the population of the United States as a whole.

Data sources: University of California, Berkeley (n.d.); authors' calculations.

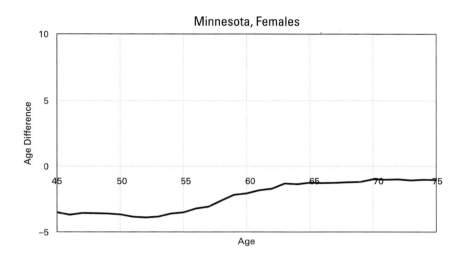

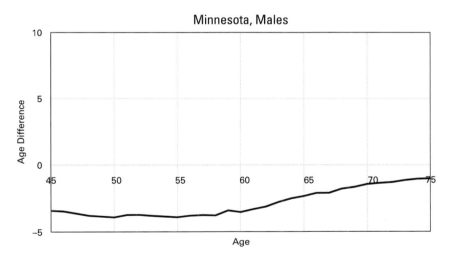

FIGURE 8.5B: Age difference trajectories for Minnesota, women and men, 2015. Standard population is the population of the United States as a whole.

Data sources: University of California, Berkeley (n.d.); authors' calculations.

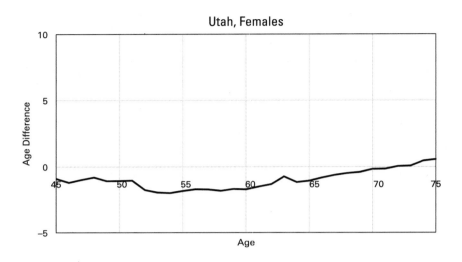

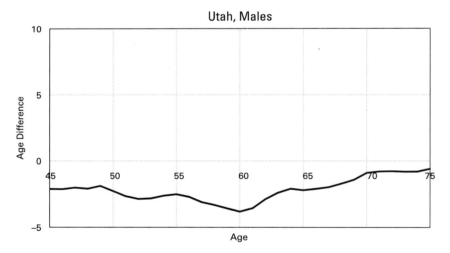

FIGURE 8.6A: Age difference trajectories for Utah, women and men, 2015. Standard population is the population of the United States as a whole.

Data sources: University of California, Berkeley (n.d.); authors' calculations.

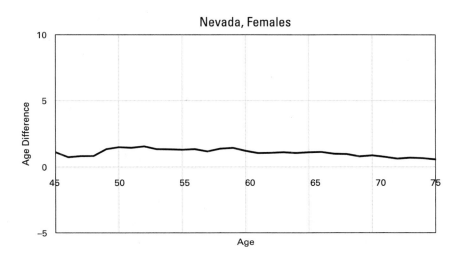

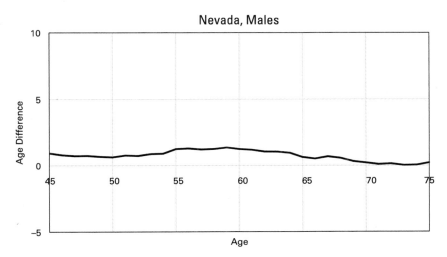

FIGURE 8.6B: Age difference trajectories for Nevada, women and men, 2015.
Standard population is the population of the United States as a whole.

Data sources: University of California, Berkeley (n.d.); authors' calculations.

is not famous for its health spas, but it is culturally different enough from Utah to make for an interesting comparison.

Figure 8.6 shows the age difference trajectories for Utah and Nevada. The age difference trajectories are roughly inverses of each other. Generally, where one is high, the other is low; where one is increasing, the other is decreasing. For example, a lifestyle without alcohol or tobacco leads 60-year-old men in Utah to have the same 10-year survival rates as men who are around 56 in the US population as a whole. In Nevada, 60-year-old men have the same survival rates as those who are around 61 years old in the United States as a whole. The effects of the lifestyle differences are less pronounced for women. In Utah, 60-year-old women have the same 10-year survival rate as 58-year-olds in the whole country, while women of that age in Nevada have the same rate as 61-year-olds.

Conclusion

We have traveled far from the familiar measures of population aging, like the *old-age dependency ratio* and the population's *median age*. The age differences and the age difference trajectories that we discussed here, unlike those older measures, are independent of the age structures of populations. Originally, age-structure-based measures conceptualized population aging as a burden; age differences and age difference trajectories do not have this orientation. Using age differences and age difference trajectories, features of population aging can now be seen that were invisible using the traditional measures. Importantly, age difference measures are a natural part of the same framework, we have been using throughout this book. *Prospective old-age thresholds (POATs), prospective old-age dependency ratios (POADRs), proportions of the 65+ population who are categorized as old (P65Os),* the *prospective proportions of adult lifetimes spent in old age (PPALOs), age differences,* and *age difference trajectories,* among other measures, are all part of our new multidimensional view of population aging.

Now that we have come so far, let's investigate what we see around us a bit more. In this chapter, we saw some interesting differences in the patterns of survival of women and men while we were walking around looking at other things. In Chapter 9, we use age difference trajectories to explore gender differences in more detail.

9

The α-Gender Gap in Survival

AFTER OUR TOUR of the Russian Federation and the United States, we have decided that Paris would be the appropriate setting to begin the next leg of our exploration. We are sitting in an outdoor café near the French Academy of Sciences enjoying a glass of wine and watching the women and men walk by. We are here because the French invented the phrase "Vive la différence." The phrase expresses the joy that the French take in exploring the differences between women and men. The origin of the phrase has been lost in history, but one, probably apocryphal, story that we have heard has it originating during a lecture by the great nineteenth-century French physiologist Claude Bernard at the Academy. While lecturing on the relatively minor physiological differences between men and women, one lively scientist is said to have shouted out "Vive la différence." In our lives, we celebrate the differences between women and men in many ways. But not all differences are something to be celebrated.

In Chapter 8, we used *age-difference trajectories* as tool for visualizing the pace of aging. Among other things, we found places where women were aging more rapidly than men. So, before we make a toast to "la différence," we use age-difference trajectories to help us better understand gender differences in survival.

Gender Gaps in Survival and Life Expectancy in Primates

In humans, women generally live longer than men. At each age, their survival rates tend to be higher. Survival rate differences between the genders are certainly influenced by social factors, but there is also an important biological component. In most other primate species for which we have data, females have higher life expectancies than males. This is true for baboons, sifaka, gorillas, chimpanzees, and capuchins (Bronikowski et al. 2011). There is also one primate species where female/male life expectancies are similar—muriquis, also known as woolly spider monkeys. What sets muriquis apart from the other primates is that males do not intensively compete with one another for mating opportunities with females. Indeed, one of the unusual features of muriquis is that males can spend time together in groups without aggressive behavior toward one another (Kemper 2013).

Human females live longer than the females of other primate species, but using the increase of mortality rates with age, Bronikowski et al. (2011) found that human females perfectly fit into the general pattern for the other primate species. Human males, on the other hand, reportedly aged more slowly than the other primate species.

In humans, gender differences in life expectancy at birth vary across space and over time. In 2015, the largest gender gap among countries of the world was in the Russian Federation (Hutt 2016). There life expectancy at birth for women was 76.3 years and 64.7 years for men. This 11.6-year gap was due largely to the unusually low life expectancy of men. At the other end of the spectrum, the lowest gender gap in life expectancy at birth in 2015 was in Mali, where it was 58.3 years for women and 58.2 years for men.

Gender Gaps in Life Expectancy in Cloistered Populations

Given this wide range of observed gender gaps in life expectancy at birth, it would be informative to find situations where the health and environmental conditions for women and men were as identical as possible and observe the life expectancy gaps in those cases. This is what was done in Luy (2003), where he analyzed the life expectancies of 11,624 Catholic nuns and monks in Bavaria from 1890 to 1995. Nuns and monks had similar daily routines, housing, diet, and medical care. They did not compete for mates or much with one another. They had no worries about who would care for them in old age or about their children. Up to the end of World War II, when some monks took up smoking while it was still prohibited for nuns, the differences in life expectancy at age 25 were small, usually well less than 1 year.

When Luy (2003) compared the increase over time in the life expectancy at age 25 of Bavarian nuns and German women in general, he found that the increases were almost identical. There was a gender gap in life expectancy of between 2 and 5 years, but that was almost entirely due to the difference between the life expectancy of German men in general and the monks. German men outside of monasteries had lower life expectancies than the monks, while German women outside of convents had about the same life expectancy as the nuns. Perhaps there is some parallel that can be drawn between the noncompetitive lifestyles of the monks and those of the woolly spider monkeys.

Daw's Measure of the Female Advantage in Survival

At each age, women tend to have higher survival rates than men. The problem with measuring the female advantage in survival is not in seeing what is around us. It is how to interpret what we see. Survival rate gaps that are large or small can both be indicative of problems. Added to the difficulty of interpreting gender differences in survival at specific ages is the additional complexity added when we wish to interpret patterns of gender gaps over ages.

One method of investigating gender gaps in survival is using ratios of death rates at the same age. Discontent with this approach was already voiced over half a century ago by Daw (1961). Daw wrote,

> The usual method of comparing male and female mortality is to use the ratio of the two death rates at the same age. This paper arose from a discontent with the ratio as a comparative measure; it was felt that behind the apparent irregularities in both time and age of the ratio there should be some sort of order or regularity which the ratio did not show up. (Daw 1961, 20)

In order to avoid the problems associated with the use of death rate ratios, Daw invented something that he called "the female advantage."
In the terminology of this book, Daw's female advantage is an *age difference*, the difference between an *α-age* and a chronological age. Female death rates were used as the *standard schedule* with which to
compute the α-ages of men.

Daw's focus was on the age difference and did not discuss α-ages.
Daw also studied how his female advantage measure changed over age
and time. The result was, to our knowledge, the first use of what we
now call *age difference trajectories*, the relationship between age differences, on the one hand, and chronological ages on the other.

To compute his female advantage, Daw first chose a particular age
and found the 1-year death rate of men at that age. Next, he found the
age of women who had the same 1-year death rate. Daw's measure of
the female advantage is the difference between the age of women and
the age of men with the same 1-year death rate.

In Table 9.1, we reproduce some of the female advantage figures (in
years) in Daw's table 1.

In reading Table 9.1, we see, for example, that, in 1841–1845, women
in England and Wales had the same 1-year death rate at age 54.8
(= 52.5 + 2.3) as men did at age 52.5. The death rate of the women rose to
the same level as observed for 52.5-year-old men when they were
2.3 years older. The advantage that the women had over 52.5-year-old
men in 1841–1845 was, therefore, 2.3 years. Two interesting features of

Table 9.1   Daw's female advantage, England and Wales

| Year | Age of men | | | |
	52.5	62.5	72.5	82.5
1841–1845	2.3	1.7	1.5	1.0
1861–1865	3.2	1.8	1.1	0.8
1881–1885	3.8	2.2	1.8	1.1
1901–1905	4.1	3.5	2.5	1.4
1921–1925	3.6	3.5	2.7	2.1
1941–1945	5.5	5.0	3.0	2.7
1951–1955	6.0	5.9	4.0	2.3

Source: Extracted from Daw (1961, 23, table 1).

the table are (1) the tendency for the female advantage to increase over time, and (2) the tendency for the female advantage to diminish with increasing age.

Not only did Daw compute female advantages over time and age groups for England and Wales, he also computed age difference trajectories in 1953–1955 for Sweden, the Netherlands, Australia, the United States (white population), England and Wales, Israel (Jewish population), Canada, France, Japan, the United States (nonwhite population), the Federal Republic of Germany, the Democratic Republic of Germany, Sri Lanka, and Mauritius (countries listed as in Daw 1961, 27, table 4).

In addition, Daw computed the female advantage using data for Roman Catholic nuns and monks in the United States involved in educational work, by causes of death, using proportions of populations surviving to specific ages, and rates of illness. Daw also showed that the female advantage in England and Wales would be more constant if age were measured from the end of life instead of the beginning.

Until we wrote this book, we were unaware of Daw's paper. After reading it, we did a search for citations to it in the bibliographic database "The Web of Science" (Thomson Reuters, n.d.). That database catalogs a vast array of articles written since the end of the nineteenth century and keeps track of all articles that have cited each paper. As of this writing, Daw's paper has been cited only twice, once in 1964 and once in 1986. We hope our book will draw more attention to Daw's pioneering work.

The Problem with Interpreting Gender Gaps in Survival

Daw criticized the literature on gender gaps in survival that preceded his research because it was based on ratios of male-to-female death rates at specific ages, but regardless of how it is done, the direct comparisons of male and female death rates suffer from a problem of interpretability. Let's take the case of the age-specific ratios of male-to-female death rates, for example. If those ratios are high, women have a large advantage in survival. That large advantage could arise because women have death rates similar to those of women in comparable countries and men have much higher death rates relative to men in those countries. Thus, a high survival advantage for women could be the result of very poor health behaviors on the part of men. The same large advantage in survival could also arise when men have death rates similar to those in comparable countries, but women have much lower ones. Thus, the same gender gap in survival could be due to relatively poor health for men or relatively good health for women. This ambiguity also arises when changes in the gender gap in survival is studied over time. The survival advantage of women could increase with the passage of time because of improving health conditions for women, deteriorating health conditions for men, or some combination of the two. To increase what we can learn from gender gap measures, it is important to supplement them with information about the survival conditions of women and men separately.

α-Gender Gaps in Survival: Methodology

Gender gaps in survival are often measured using ratios of mortality rates (MPIDR, n.d.), but, as we discussed, what we see with these ratios is difficult to interpret. We aim to provide a broader framework for the studying of gender differences in survival, one which provides an integrated view of those gender differences and the context in which they are embedded. The gender gaps that we investigate in this chapter are gender gaps in 5-year survival rates, although all the figures that we produce would be exactly the same if we used 5-year death rates instead. To see gender gaps more clearly, we use age differences, the differences between α-ages and chronological ages. To distinguish the gender gaps that we see from the more traditional ones, we call them *α-gender gaps*.

Context is important in interpreting gender differences in survival. We provide it by producing two age difference trajectories, one for women and one for men. The calculation of those age difference trajectories requires two standard populations. We use women and men in Japan as the standard populations. During the period 1980–1985 to 2010–2015, Japanese women had the highest life expectancy at birth among all female populations for which the United Nations produced life tables. Japanese men did not always have the top life expectancy but were always close to the best. The age differences provide context because they are relative to a country with the highest or close to the highest survival rates. The age differences, then, show how far the 5-year survival rates are from the world champion for women and a near world champion for men. α-gender gaps, then, are computed as differences in how far each gender is behind the best or nearly best survival rates in the world.

Because our interest is in population aging, we focus here on ages 45 and 75 and two time periods, 1980–1985 and 2010–2015. The period 2010–2015 is the most recent period for which estimated (as opposed to projected) life tables are available from the United Nations (2017e). We go back 30 years because that matches the 30-year age span, from age 45 to age 75, that we study.

The first step in computing α-gender gaps in survival is the calculation of gender-specific age differences. In Table 9.2, we show the age differences for Australian men. The table can be read in three ways: (1) reading across the rows, holds the year constant, and shows the age differences at different ages; (2) reading down a column holds age constant and shows us how age differences looked in different years; (3) the table can also be read on a diagonal. The survivors of people who were 45 in 1980–1985 were 75 in 2010–2015.

In 1980–1985, the age difference for Australian men was 0.4 years. In other words, 45-year-old Australian men in 1980–1985 had the same 5-year survival rate as 45.4-year-old Japanese men in that year. In 2010–2015, the age difference was 0. In 2010–2015, 45-year-old Australian men had the same 5-year survival rate as 45-year-old Japanese men in the same time period. Survival rates increased from 1980–1985 to

Table 9.2   Age differences for Australia, using Japanese life tables for the indicated year as standards

	Males	
Age	45	75
Year		
1980–1985	0.4	1.2
2010–2015	0.0	−0.3

Data sources: United Nations (2017e); authors' calculations.

2010–2015 for both Japanese and Australian men. They increased slightly faster for Australian men resulting in a decrease in the age difference. In 1980–1985, 75-year-old Australian men had an age difference of 1.2 years. The age difference for 45-year-old men in 1980–1985 was 0.4, so 75-year-old men in 1980–1985 were slightly further behind the Japanese than were 45-year-old men at the time. In 2010–2015, the age difference for Japanese men was –0.3 years. In other words, the 5-year survival rate for Australian 75-year-old men was the same as 74.7-year-old Japanese men in that year.

Between 1980–1985 and 2010–2015, we observe that the age difference fell from 0.4 to 0.0 for 45-year-old men and from 1.2 to –0.3 for 75-year-olds. Relative to the Japanese, survival rates fell more rapidly for the 75-year-old men, when age is assessed using 5-year survival rates as the characteristic of interest. We see the same thing when we take a longitudinal perspective. In 1980–1985, 45-year-old men had an age difference of 0.4 years. Their survivors 30 years later had an age difference of –0.3 years. In terms of 5-year survival rates, in 1980–1985, Australian men were slightly behind their Japanese counterparts, and 30 years later, those who survived were slightly ahead. The age differences in Table 9.2 are not large. The broad message of the table is that from 1980–1985 to 2010–2015, Australian men were aging similarly to the Japanese men.

We have produced tables like 9.2 for each gender and for a variety of countries. They are the raw materials that we use in the computation of α-gender gaps in survival.

α-Gender Gaps in Survival: Example

In Table 9.3, we illustrate the computation of α-gender gaps by continuing our Australian example.

In Table 9.3, the data for men are the same as in Table 9.2, and they are supplemented with two additional elements, the history for women and the α-gender gap. We see that the age difference for 45-year-old Australian women in 1980–1985 was 2.4 years. This means that 45-year-old Australian women in 1980–1985 had the same 5-year survival rate as 47.4-year-old Japanese women in the same time period. In 1980–1985, 45-year-old Australian men had the same 5-year survival rates as

Table 9.3 α-gender gaps in Australia, using Japanese populations as standards

	45			75		
	Male	Female	Gap	Male	Female	Gap
Year						
1980–1985	0.4	2.4	−2.0	1.2	0.1	1.1
2010–2015	0.0	1.4	−1.4	−0.3	1.9	−2.3

Data sources: United Nations (2017c); authors' calculations.

45.4-year-old Japanese men. So 45-year-old Australian women were further behind Japanese women than 45-year-old Australian men were behind Japanese men.

We compute the α-gender gap as the difference between the male age difference and the female age difference. Age differences are measured in years, so the difference is also measured in terms of years. In this case, the α-gender gap in survival for 45-year-old Australians in 1980–1985 was −2.0 years. In all our gender gap calculations, a negative α-gender gap indicates a gender gap to the disadvantage of women. A positive α-gender gap indicates a gender gap to the disadvantage of men. A gender gap of 0 indicates no gender gap relative to the Japanese standard population. Whether computations were arranged so that a negative α-gender gap indicated a gap to the disadvantage of women or to the disadvantage of men is of no consequence here. Crucial is that, even though women generally have higher survival rates than men at each age, there can still be gender gaps to their disadvantage. The gender gap compares how far women are behind Japanese women to how far men are behind Japanese men. If women in a country are further behind their Japanese counterparts than men in the country, then there is an α-gender gap in survival to their disadvantage.

When we look at age 45, we see that from 1980–1985 to 2010–2015, the age difference for both Australian women and men fell. Survival rates were converging toward those of the Japanese for both genders. The decline in the age difference was greater for women than for men and because of this, the α-gender gap to the disadvantage of women decreased, going from −2.0 in 1980–1985 to −1.4 in 2010–2015.

The picture at age 75 is different. The α-gender gap in 1980–1985 was 1.1, indicating a small α-gender gap to the disadvantage of men. Between 1980–1985 and 2010–2015, the survival rates of Australian men moved downward toward those of Japanese men and survival rates for Australian women moved upward relative to those in Japan. The result was a change in direction of the α-gender gap, from one that was to the disadvantage of men in 1980–1985 to one that was to the disadvantage of women in 2010–2015.

α-Gender Gaps in Survival: Observations

Now that we have gone through an example of how to read our gender gap tables, let us look around and see what the world looks like from this perspective. We do this using a set of country comparisons, each with a table like the one above for Australia. Our goal is to discover whether there are interesting regional or global patterns. At the end of our tour, we would like to have accumulated evidence on whether α-gender gaps in survival have generally been diminishing over time.

In Table 9.4, we show a comparison of Poland and the Russian Federation. In 1980–1985, 45-year-old Russian men had the same 5-year survival rates as 59.2-year-old Japanese men in that year. Relative to Japanese men, the survival rate of 45-year-old Russian men deteriorated over time. In 2010–2015, 45-year-old Russian men had the same 5-year

Table 9.4   α-gender gaps for Poland and the Russian Federation, using Japanese populations as standards

	45			75		
	Male	Female	Difference	Male	Female	Difference
Poland						
1980–1985	8.1	5.6	2.5	3.2	2.8	0.4
2010–2015	9.6	5.7	3.9	3.9	4.8	−0.8
Russian Federation						
1980–1985	14.2	9.1	5.1	3.9	3.1	0.8
2010–2015	17.5	14.7	2.8	6.9	8.2	−1.3

Data sources: United Nations (2017e); authors' calculations.

Note: Numbers are rounded independently.

survival rate as 62.5-year-old Japanese men. For both genders and for both ages, we observe a relative deterioration between 1980–1985 and 2010–2015. At age 45, the α-gender gap was to the disadvantage of men and was smaller at both ages in 2010–2015 than in 1980–1985. This was due to the larger deterioration for women than for men. At age 75, the larger deterioration for women turned a small α-gender gap to the disadvantage of men into a small gap to the disadvantage of women.

We also see a deterioration in relative survival conditions between 1980–1985 and 2010–2015 in Poland. In contrast to the case of the Russian Federation, the α-gender gap at age 45 shows an increase in the disadvantage for men. This was largely due to the differences in the changes in relative survival rates for women. In the Russian Federation, there was a comparatively large deterioration for women, while in Poland the change was only one-tenth of a year. In Poland, as in the Russian Federation, a small α-gender gap to the disadvantage of men at age 75 in 1980–1985 turned into a small α-gender gap to the disadvantage of women in 2010–2015.

In Table 9.5, we compare Australia and the United States. We already discussed the Australian observations above. When we looked at Poland and the Russian Federation, we observed a relative decline in survival rates for both genders and at both ages. This is not what we see for Australia. For both genders at age 45 and for men at age 75, we see the age differences in the table moving closer to 0 (the levels for

Table 9.5 α-gender gaps for Australia and the United States, using Japanese populations as standards

	45			75		
	Male	Female	Difference	Male	Female	Difference
Australia						
1980–1985	0.4	2.4	−2.0	1.2	0.1	1.1
2010–2015	0.0	1.4	−1.4	−0.3	1.9	−2.3
United States						
1980–1985	3.0	4.9	−1.8	0.3	−0.4	0.1
2010–2015	5.7	8.7	−3.0	1.1	4.2	−3.1

Data sources: United Nations (2017e); authors' calculations.

Note: Numbers are rounded independently.

the Japanese) over time. In contrast to the observation for Australia, but like Poland and the Russian Federation, in the United States we observe a generalized relative deterioration over time, as all the age differences are larger in 2010–2015 than in 1980–1985. In the United States, there was already an α-gender gap to the disadvantage of women for 45-year-old women in 1980–1985 and it became larger over time because the relative survival rate of 45-year-old women decreased more than for men of the same age. An α-gender gap to the disadvantage of 75-year-old women opened up in 2010–2015 for the same reasons.

In Table 9.6, we compare China with Hong Kong. All the numbers in the table for Hong Kong are comparatively small, so the people in Hong Kong were aging much like the people in Japan. At age 45 in 1980–1985, the 5-year survival rate of 45-year-old Chinese women was the same as 52.4-year-old Japanese women in that year; while 45-year-old Chinese men had the same 5-year survival rate as 46.4-year-old Japanese men. The result was an almost 6-year α-gender gap to the disadvantage of women in China at age 45 in 1980–1985. The α-gender gap to the disadvantage of 45-year-old women was smaller in 2010–2015. The age difference for 45-year-old men was larger than it was in 1980–1985 and the one for women was smaller. For 75-year-olds, the α-gender gap to the disadvantage of women was larger in 2010–2015 than it had been in 1980–1985. Relatively, survival rates were further from the Japanese standards in 2010–2015, and the relative deterioration was larger for women.

Table 9.6 α-gender gaps for China and Hong Kong, using Japanese populations as standards

	45			75		
	Male	Female	Difference	Male	Female	Difference
China						
1980–1985	1.4	7.4	−5.9	4.1	5.1	−1.0
2010–2015	1.8	5.3	−3.4	6.1	9.2	−3.1
Hong Kong						
1980–1985	1.0	1.9	−0.9	0.6	0.2	0.4
2010–2015	−0.9	−0.9	0.0	0.2	1.2	−0.9

Data sources: United Nations (2017e); authors' calculations.
Note: Numbers are rounded independently.

Table 9.7 compares France and the United Kingdom. In France, the α-gender gaps are all to the disadvantage of men, except for 75-year-olds in 2010–2015. In the United Kingdom, the α-gender gaps are all to the disadvantage of women except for 75-year-olds in 1980–1985. The largest α-gender gaps in the table are observed in the United Kingdom at age 45 in 1980–1985 and at age 75 in 2010–2015. They were to the disadvantage of women and were largely due to the relatively low survival rates of women at those ages.

Our next comparison in Table 9.8 is between Kenya and South Africa. Between 1980–1985 and 2010–2015, South Africa was significantly

Table 9.7   α-gender gaps for France and the United Kingdom, using Japanese populations as standards

	45			75		
	Male	Female	Difference	Male	Female	Difference
France						
1980–1985	4.6	2.9	1.7	0.9	−0.1	1.0
2010–2015	4.2	3.4	0.7	−0.2	0.8	−1.0
United Kingdom						
1980–1985	0.6	3.7	−3.1	2.5	1.4	1.1
2010–2015	1.3	3.0	−1.8	0.7	3.7	−3.0

Data sources: United Nations (2017e); authors' calculations.
Note: Numbers are rounded independently.

Table 9.8   α-gender gaps for Kenya and South Africa, using Japanese populations as standards

	45			75		
	Male	Female	Difference	Male	Female	Difference
Kenya						
1980–1985	9.8	14.7	−4.9	2.6	4.8	−2.2
2010–2015	16.0	20.8	−4.8	5.7	10.5	−4.8
South Africa						
1980–1985	15.4	17.2	−1.8	6.0	5.5	0.5
2010–2015	24.2	26.2	−1.9	8.9	9.9	−1.1

Data sources: United Nations (2017e); authors' calculations.
Note: Numbers are rounded independently.

Table 9.9   α-gender gaps for Cuba and Puerto Rico, using Japanese
populations as standards

	45			75		
	Male	Female	Difference	Male	Female	Difference
Cuba						
1980–1985	0.9	5.9	−5.0	−1.5	0.4	−2.0
2010–2015	4.4	7.0	−2.7	1.7	5.0	−3.2
Puerto Rico						
1980–1985	8.0	4.5	3.5	−1.7	0.2	−1.9
2010–2015	8.0	3.5	4.5	2.5	3.8	−1.3

Data sources: United Nations (2017e); authors' calculations.
Note: Numbers are rounded independently.

affected by the HIV pandemic. Kenya was much less affected. Nevertheless, we see substantial deteriorations in relative survival rates in
both countries. In Kenya, there were larger gender gaps to the disadvantage of women. This was not mainly due to differences in relative
survival rates for women. The main reason for the larger α-gender gap
to the disadvantage of women in Kenya was the relatively higher 5-year
survival rates of Kenyan men compared with South African men.

Our final comparison is between Cuba and Puerto Rico. One interesting feature of Table 9.9 is the comparison between female and male
survival rates for 45-year-olds in Puerto Rico. There we see a comparatively large α-gender gap to the disadvantage of men. In Cuba, α-gender
gaps were all to the disadvantage of women.

Conclusion

We have wandered through the complex environment of α-gender gaps in
survival and looked at its topographic features from a new perspective.
We began by asking whether we would find α-gender gaps decreasing
over time. We did not find this. Instead, we found a wide variety of patterns but little global consistency. Even though, women generally
have higher survival rates than men, we found that there were often
α-gender gaps in survival to their disadvantage and that there was no
consistent pattern of those gaps decreasing over time.

We saw many intriguing features but that is far from explaining them. The case of the relatively low survival rates of 45-year-old Puerto Rican men is an interesting example of this. Those relatively low survival rates could be due to migration. It is possible that healthier males are more likely to migrate to the mainland of the United States than healthier females. Alternatively, there might be some parallel between the situation in Eastern Europe and Puerto Rico. Perhaps the lack of economic opportunities for Puerto Rican men compared to their expectations resulted in depression and poor health behaviors.

This chapter introduces the idea of thinking about "la différence" in survival not in terms of some direct comparison between women and men but in a two-step process where women and men are first compared to cases of best practice for their genders. If women were further behind best practice than men, there would be an α-gender gap to the disadvantage of women. If men were further behind best practice, there would be an α-gender gap to the disadvantage of men.

The methodological problem is how to do this in a way that yields results that are interpretable and not sensitive to irrelevant changes in how characteristics are measured. Our approach of relating characteristics to ages meets these goals. α-gender gaps are measured in years. If the α-gender gap is 2 years, for example, it means that men are 2 years further behind best practice than are women. An advantage of translating characteristics into ages is that it is insensitive to the metric used to quantify the characteristic. We discussed the details of this in the appendix to Chapter 5. In the context of this chapter, this means that all the results are the same regardless of whether we use death rates or survival rates. We studied α-gender gaps using 5-year survival rates as a characteristic. However, our approach is more general and could employ many different characteristics, including activity limitations and self-rated health.

Now that we have spent a while in the less familiar terrain of age difference measures and α-gender gaps, it is time to return to the more familiar territory of *prospective old-age dependency ratios (POADRs)* and *prospective median ages (PMAs)*. In Chapter 10, we aim to answer the question, What will happen to measures of population aging if there is a scientific breakthrough that slows the aging process in humans?

10

What Would Happen to Population Aging If Life Expectancy Increase Sped Up?

IN 2014, Joon Yun, president of Palo Alto Investors, LLC offered $1 million in prize money for cutting-edge research on increasing human longevity. Yun is a radiologist whose firm manages over $2 billion of assets invested in the healthcare industry. He now presides over two Palo Alto Longevity Prizes each worth half a million dollars. According to the website for the Palo Alto Longevity Prize,

> A $500,000 Homeostatic Capacity Prize will be awarded to the first team to demonstrate that it can restore homeostatic capacity (using heart rate variability as the surrogate measure) of an aging reference mammal to that of a young adult. . . .
>
> A $500,000 Longevity Demonstration Prize will be awarded to the first Team that meets all the requirements . . . including extending the mean lifespan of a wild-type mammalian intervention cohort by 50% relative to acceptable published natural history of untreated norms in a statistically significant ($p < .05$) manner. (Race Against Time Foundation 2017)

The Palo Alto Longevity Prizes are only the tip of a very large iceberg of aging research done at companies, universities, and research institutes across the globe. Ben Kamens's Spring Discovery is also in Silicon Valley. According to the Spring Discovery website,

We've built a machine learning platform to accelerate experimentation for discovering therapies for aging and its related diseases.

While the science of aging research is full of promising results, it still takes far too long to run experiments. This significantly slows down the search for therapies that could one day reduce cardiovascular disease, neurodegenerative diseases, arthritis, and more. Spring Discovery's machine learning-based experimentation platform solves this. We're applying a novel computational approach to one of the most important problems in the world: battling aging and disease. (Spring Discovery, n.d.)

A bit farther north, in South San Francisco, Google set up a company called Calico to develop new ways of increasing longevity (Wikipedia, n.d.a). The quest to lengthen life is an old one and a breakthrough could be right around the corner. A drug that has quadrupled the lifespan of a strain of mice is already being tested on people and the president of the organization administering the Palo Alto Longevity Prizes thinks that a lifespan of 120 healthy years might be attainable in the near term (Wong 2016). It also might be that eating broccoli and exercising regularly could remain the best ways to extend longevity for many decades to come. We just don't know.

Longevity in the future could be quite different from what we would expect from a projection of what we have observed over the last century. So, we flew over to Silicon Valley in California. It is a good place to begin an exploration of what could happen if their efforts to increase life expectancy succeeded.

We begin by looking at what others have said about the apparently innocuous question: What causes population aging? The consensus view is stated in a joint World Health Organization and US National Institute of Aging report:

In 2010, an estimated 524 million people were 65 or older—8 percent of the world's population. By 2050, this number is expected to nearly triple to about 1.5 billion, representing 16 percent of the world's population. . . . This remarkable phenomenon is being driven by declines in fertility and improvements in longevity. (WHO and US National Institute of Aging 2011, 4)

A more nuanced assessment can be found in *World Population Ageing 2015:*

> As fertility rates fall over time, the size of birth cohorts stabilizes and improvements in longevity become increasingly important drivers of population ageing. (United Nations 2015, 48)

Wikipedia, seemingly the most trusted source of information among college students, provides this definition:

> Population ageing is an increasing median age in the population of a region due to declining fertility rates and/or rising life expectancy. (Wikipedia, n.d.c)

The consensus assessment that population aging is due to the fall in fertility and increases in longevity is repeated in scores of journal articles, reports, and websites. In a world where the *proportion of the population categorized as being old (PO)* is the proportion 65 years old or older, this conclusion is undeniable. A fall in fertility, other things being equal, decreases the number of young people but not the number of people aged 65 and over, and, therefore, increases the PO. An increase in life expectancy at age 65, other things being equal, increases the number of those 65-year-olds, but does not change the number of younger people, and, therefore, also increases the PO. Increases in longevity coupled with decreasing or constant fertility will cause the PO to increase. The conclusion is clear. The research of people who win the Palo Alto Longevity Prize could eventually lead to a large increase in population aging. Should we worry that the success of scientific studies devoted to slowing aging could eventually backfire and leave populations worse off because of the induced age structure change?

Making Population Forecasts Using Three Speeds of Life Expectancy Increase

To investigate the effects of increases in longevity on aging, we would need data on how measures of aging evolved when life expectancy change was slower and when it was faster. Naturally, there are no observations on countries where, in one reality, longevity increases were slower and, in another, everything was the same except that longevity increases were faster. But just because we cannot observe these different realities does not mean that we cannot simulate them on our computers. In the European Demographic Data Sheet (VID and IIASA 2016), population forecasts were made for 43 European countries for the period of 2015 to 2050. For us, the simplest way to assess the effects of the speed of life expectancy change on measures of population aging was to rerun those forecasts, changing only the pace of life expectancy improvement. So, the differences that we observe in measures of population aging are due to differences in the speed of life expectancy increase and nothing else.

For simplicity, we ran three scenarios for each country. Scenario 3 was the forecast that appeared in VID and IIASA (2016). It was the forecast that we considered to be the most likely. In scenario 3, life expectancy at birth generally increased by around 2 years per decade. In scenario 2, life expectancy increased half as fast as it was in scenario 3. In scenario 1, there was no life expectancy increase over the 35-year period, so age-specific survival rates were the same in 2050 as they were in 2015. For the 43 countries listed in the European Demographic Data Sheet 2016, for all three scenarios, and for the years 2015, 2030, and 2050, we calculated *old-age dependency ratios (OADR), prospective old-age dependency ratios (POADR), median ages (MA),* and *prospective median ages (PMA)*. Table 10.1 is an example of the tables that we produced comparing changes in the OADR and the POADR using data for Armenia, a country in Europe that we have not visited so far.

In Armenia, the OADR increases from 0.17 in 2015 to 0.42 in 2050 in scenario 3. In scenario 1, all the elements of the population forecast are the same except that there is no increase in life expectancy. In scenario 1, the OADR increases from 0.17 in 2015 to 0.35 in 2050. The column labeled "Difference" is the difference between the OADRs in scenario 3 and scenario 1. The difference between scenario 2 and scenario 1 is about half as large. The figures in that column show the effects of faster increases in life expectancy. The positive figures in the column show that, when life expectancy increase is faster, the increase in the OADR is also faster. This is what we discussed above. Faster increases in life expectancy, taken by themselves, are associated with faster increases in conventional measures of aging.

Table 10.1 Prospective and conventional old-age dependency ratios for three scenarios of life expectancy increase, Armenia, 2015, 2030, and 2050

	Old-age dependency ratio				Prospective old-age dependency ratio			
	Scen. 1	Scen. 2	Scen. 3	Difference	Scen. 1	Scen. 2	Scen. 3	Difference
2015	0.17	0.17	0.17		0.16	0.16	0.16	
2030	0.29	0.30	0.30	0.01	0.26	0.24	0.22	−0.04
2050	0.35	0.38	0.42	0.08	0.31	0.27	0.24	−0.07

Data sources: VID and IIASA (2016); authors' calculations.
Note: Scenario 1 assumes no life expectancy increase. Scenario 3 assumes the same life expectancy increase as in the European Demographic Data Sheet 2016, and scenario 2 assumes half as much increase in life expectancy as in scenario 3. The number under "Difference" is the difference between scenario 3 and scenario 1. Numbers are rounded independently.

When we look at the effects of faster increases of life expectancy on the POADR, we see something different. In scenario 3, the POADR increases from 0.16 in 2015 to 0.24 in 2050. The difference between scenario 2 and scenario 1 is again about half as large. Armenia is aging because of past age structure changes, but the increase in the POADR is much slower than the increase in the OADR. We showed other examples of this general result in Chapter 4. Most importantly, the differences are negative, indicating that when the POADR is used to assess population aging faster increases in life expectancy lead to slower aging.

The Speed of Aging and the Speed of Life Expectancy Change: Old-Age Dependency Ratios

Using the analogue of Table 10.1 for each of the 43 countries in the European Demographic Data Sheet 2016, we focused on the two most important numbers, those for scenario 3 and scenario 1 in 2050. Using the OADR, that number in Table 10.1 is 0.08, and using the POADR, it is −0.07. In Table 10.2, we show the corresponding numbers for all the countries.

In each country the sign of the difference is positive when population aging is measured using the OADR and negative when using the POADR. We present data for 43 countries here to demonstrate that the observation that faster life expectancy increases lead to slower population aging when the POADR is used is the case for a wide variety of demographic regimes.

The Speed of Aging and the Speed of Life Expectancy Change: Median Ages

We also see that faster increases in life expectancy lead to slower population aging when population aging is assessed using changes in the MA. Table 10.3 shows the effects of faster life expectancy increases on the MA and on the PMA of the Armenian population. The computation of PMA requires that we specify a life expectancy schedule as a standard. For each country in the European Data Sheet 2016, we take each country's life expectancy schedule (both sexes combined) in 2015

Table 10.2 Differences between scenario 3 and scenario 1 in 2050 using the old-age dependency ratio and the prospective old-age dependency ratio, 43 European countries

	Old-age dependency ratio difference	Prospective old-age dependency ratio difference
Albania	0.08	−0.03
Armenia	0.08	−0.07
Austria	0.09	−0.03
Azerbaijan	0.07	−0.06
Belarus	0.09	−0.08
Belgium	0.08	−0.03
Bulgaria	0.10	−0.07
Croatia	0.13	−0.07
Cyprus	0.09	−0.04
Czech Republic	0.10	−0.07
Denmark	0.08	−0.03
Estonia	0.10	−0.06
Finland	0.09	−0.03
France	0.09	−0.03
Georgia	0.08	−0.07
Germany	0.11	−0.03
Greece	0.13	−0.07
Hungary	0.10	−0.07
Iceland	0.08	−0.03
Ireland	0.09	−0.06
Italy	0.12	−0.06
Latvia	0.09	−0.06
Lithuania	0.10	−0.03
Luxembourg	0.06	−0.03
Macedonia	0.09	−0.07
Malta	0.09	−0.05
Moldova	0.08	−0.12
Montenegro	0.08	−0.06
Netherlands	0.10	−0.03
Norway	0.07	−0.03
Poland	0.09	−0.06
Portugal	0.13	−0.07
Romania	0.09	−0.06
Russian Federation	0.06	−0.07
Serbia	0.10	−0.06
Slovakia	0.11	−0.09
Slovenia	0.12	−0.06
Spain	0.12	−0.08
Sweden	0.07	−0.03
Switzerland	0.09	−0.03
Turkey	0.06	−0.05
United Kingdom	0.08	−0.03
Ukraine	0.08	−0.09

Data sources: VID and IIASA (2016); authors' calculations.

Note: Scenario 1 assumes no life expectancy increase. Scenario 3 assumes the same life expectancy increase as in the European Demographic Data Sheet 2016. The number under "Difference" is the difference between scenario 3 and scenario 1.

Table 10.3 Prospective and conventional median ages for three scenarios of life expectancy increase, Armenia, 2015, 2030, and 2050

	Median age				Prospective median age			
	Scen. 1	Scen. 2	Scen. 3	Difference	Scen. 1	Scen. 2	Scen. 3	Difference
2015	34.0	34.0	34.0		34.0	34.0	34.0	
2030	40.3	40.5	40.6	0.3	40.3	39.2	38.0	−2.3
2050	42.9	44.0	45.3	2.4	42.9	41.0	39.1	−3.7

Data sources: VID and IIASA (2016); authors' calculations.
Note: Scenario 1 assumes no life expectancy increase. Scenario 3 assumes the same life expectancy increase as in the European Demographic Data Sheet 2016. The number under "Difference" is the difference between scenario 3 and scenario 1.

as the standard. In particular, when computing the PMA of the Armenian population, we take Armenian life expectancy schedule in 2015 as its standard. This is the reason why the MA and the PMA in 2015 are the same.

In the European Demographic Data Sheet 2016, we see that the MA of Armenia's population is forecast to increase by 11.3 years, from 34.0 to 45.3, from 2015 to 2050. These numbers are those in scenario 3. When population aging is measured using changes in the PMA, we see an increase of only 5.1 years, from 34.0 in 2015 to 39.1 in 2050. Next we look at the effect of faster increases in life expectancy. In scenario 1, when there is no life expectancy increase between 2015 and 2050, the MA of Armenia's population in 2050 is forecasted to be 42.9. When the forecasted increase in life expectancy is included, the MA rises to 45.3. But when population aging is gauged using the PMA, we see something different: faster growth in life expectancy results in slower aging. The PMA in scenario 3 is less than in scenario 1.

In Table 10.4, we show the differences between scenario 3 and scenario 1 in 2050 for the same countries as in Table 10.2.

In Table 10.4, as in Table 10.2, every number in the left column is positive and every number in the right column is negative. Unlike what we see when our vision was restricted to measures of population aging based solely on chronological age, when prospective measures of aging are used, faster increases in life expectancy result in slower aging. This observation is quite general. In this chapter, we observed it in simulations of a variety of European countries with quite different age structures. In Ediev, Sanderson, and Scherbov (2019), we have complemented the simulations presented here with a formal mathematical model, which explains why faster life expectancy increases are likely to lead to slower population aging (using prospective measures) all over the world in the future.

Conclusion

Let us step back from all the numbers for a moment and consider what it means for faster increases in longevity to lead to slower population aging. Prizes like the Palo Alto Longevity Prizes are for research that slows the aging process. The prize is not for finding a pill that given,

Table 10.4 Differences between scenario 3 and scenario 1 in 2050 using the median age and the prospective median age, 43 European countries

	Median age difference	Prospective median age difference
Albania	2.0	−3.9
Armenia	2.4	−3.7
Austria	2.3	−4.1
Azerbaijan	1.9	−4.2
Belarus	3.3	−3.1
Belgium	1.9	−4.6
Bulgaria	3.0	−3.2
Croatia	3.6	−2.8
Cyprus	2.1	−4.5
Czech Republic	2.6	−4.0
Denmark	2.1	−4.5
Estonia	2.9	−3.4
Finland	2.2	−4.3
France	2.1	−4.4
Georgia	3.2	−2.8
Germany	2.7	−3.8
Greece	3.1	−3.3
Hungary	3.0	−3.6
Iceland	2.0	−4.6
Ireland	1.8	−4.6
Italy	2.6	−3.9
Latvia	2.8	−3.5
Lithuania	3.4	−2.9
Luxembourg	1.5	−5.2
Macedonia	2.7	−3.5
Malta	2.4	−4.0
Moldova	3.2	−3.0
Montenegro	2.3	−4.1
Netherlands	2.3	−4.1
Norway	1.7	−4.9
Poland	2.8	−3.6
Portugal	2.9	−3.5
Romania	2.6	−3.7
Russian Federation	2.3	−3.9
Serbia	2.6	−3.7
Slovakia	3.4	−2.9
Slovenia	3.4	−3.1
Spain	2.8	−3.7
Sweden	1.8	−4.7
Switzerland	2.2	−4.3
Turkey	1.5	−4.5
United Kingdom	2.0	−4.6
Ukraine	2.8	−3.2

Data sources: VID and IIASA (2016); authors' calculations.

Note: Scenario 1 assumes no life expectancy increase. Scenario 3 assumes the same life expectancy increase as in the European Demographic Data Sheet 2016. The number under "Difference" is the difference between scenario 3 and scenario 1.

for example, to 70-year-olds with all their accumulated health deficits, allows them to live more years. The research is to slow aging so that 70-year-olds in the future will have the health, stamina, cognitive abilities, and a wide set of other characteristics more like those of perhaps 50-year-olds sometime in the past. Therefore, life expectancy improvements do not translate into more aging, because 70-year-olds in the future will not be like 70-year-olds today, especially if scientific breakthroughs slow aging. But this possibility cannot be seen when we wear the old, one-dimensional glasses. With one-dimensional vision slowing individual aging can only be seen as increasing population aging.

In this chapter, we used three scenarios to look at what would happen in the future if life expectancy increased at different speeds. The fastest speed that we envisioned was the one that we had predicted (VID and IIASA 2016). We found that the faster life expectancy increased the slower populations aged. We do not know how people will age in the future, but we find little to fear at the prospect of faster life expectancy increase.

Even without amazing breakthroughs, the United Nations forecasts life expectancy at older ages to continue rising. If that is the case, are we already living in a world of eternal aging? Will we see populations just continue to grow older and older? We answer these questions in Chapter 11.

11

If Life Expectancy Continues to Increase, Will Population Aging Ever Stop?

WHAT DOES OUR long-term future look like if life expectancy continues to increase? Will we be living in an eternally aging world? The infirmities of old age will not vanish. The human life cycle, from birth to growth to maturity to old age, will always be with us. But populations are not people. Populations can grow younger over time, even though every current member of the population is growing older, and populations can stop aging, even though every current member of the population is aging.

We begin this chapter by looking at the question of long-term population aging using the old glasses. The United Nations has made forecasts of life expectancy at 65 (both sexes combined) for the world. Life expectancy at age 65 in 2015–2020 is forecasted to be 16.98 years and to rise steadily to 18.99 years by 2045–2050 and to 21.82 years by 2095–2100. Figures 11.1 and 11.2 show the evolution of two conventional measures of aging, the *old-age dependency ratio* and the *median age* for the population of the world, based on data from the *United Nations' World Population Prospects: The 2017 Revision* (United Nations 2017c). Both measures show the population of the world continuing to age throughout the century. So, yes, with the old glasses on, it looks like the world's population will continue to age throughout this century and perhaps beyond. When the future is viewed through the old glasses, population aging does indeed appear to go on as far as the eye can see.

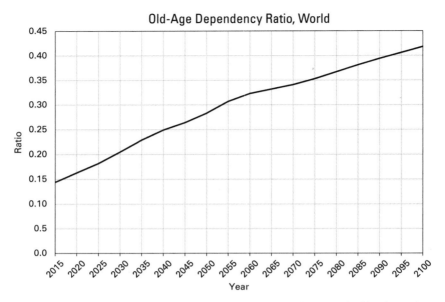

FIGURE 11.1: Old-age dependency ratio (OADR, people 65 and older/people 20–65), both sexes combined, for the world.

Data source: United Nations (2017c).

Endless Aging and the Struldbrug

To search for insights into the question of endless aging, we have been exploring islands southeast of Japan in the hope of finding the fabled island of Luggnagg. It is said that Lemuel Gulliver traveled there and learned about a small group of people called Struldbrugs (Swift 1726). Gulliver was told that most Luggnaggians live normal lifetimes, but rarely a Struldbrug is born to them. Struldbrugs live forever, but Struldbrugs do not have eternal youth.

In conversation, Gulliver finds out how difficult the life of Struldbrugs can be. This is what his acquaintance is said to have told him:

> When they came to fourscore years, which is reckoned the extremity of living in this country, they had not only all the follies and infirmities of other old men, but many more which arose from the dreadful prospect of never dying. They were not only opinionative, peevish, covetous, morose, vain, talkative, but incapable of friendship, and

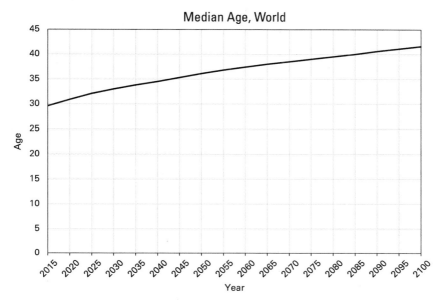

FIGURE 11.2: Median age of the world's population, both sexes combined. *Data source:* United Nations (2017c).

dead to all natural affection, which never descended below their grandchildren. Envy and impotent desires are their prevailing passions. But those objects against which their envy seems principally directed, are the vices of the younger sort and the deaths of the old. By reflecting on the former, they find themselves cut off from all possibility of pleasure; and whenever they see a funeral, they lament and repine that others have gone to a harbour of rest to which they themselves never can hope to arrive. They have no remembrance of anything but what they learned and observed in their youth and middle-age, and even that is very imperfect; and for the truth or particulars of any fact, it is safer to depend on common tradition, than upon their best recollections. The least miserable among them appear to be those who turn to dotage, and entirely lose their memories; these meet with more pity and assistance, because they want many bad qualities which abound in others. (Swift 1726, part III, chapter X)

If Gulliver had some demographic training, he may have envisioned doing a back-of-the-envelope calculation about how long it would take before most of the population of Luggnagg would all be Struldbrugs and we will not undertake such a calculation here either, as tempting as it is for us. For our purposes, it is not the suffering of the Struldbrugs that is of interest here, but how the other Luggnaggians deal with them. Gulliver is told,

> As soon as they have completed the term of eighty years, they are looked on as dead in law; their heirs immediately succeed to their estates; only a small pittance is reserved for their support; and the poor ones are maintained at the public charge. After that period, they are held incapable of any employment of trust or profit; they cannot purchase lands, or take leases; neither are they allowed to be witnesses in any cause, either civil or criminal. (Swift 1726, part III, chapter X)

It seems that Struldbrugs must surely have suffered enough. Why, then, did Luggnaggian society compound their suffering? Why couldn't older Struldbrugs coexist normally with other Luggnaggians? The answer given to Gulliver is, "As avarice is the necessary consequence of old age, those immortals would in time become proprietors of the whole nation, and engross the civil power, which, for want of abilities to manage, must end in the ruin of the public" (Swift 1726, part III, chapter X).

Struldbrugs, it turns out, were feared by other Luggnaggians. Their fear was that the Struldbrugs would inevitably acquire too much wealth and power and that they would use their wealth and power unwisely, because they did not have the mental capacity to do otherwise.

In the world of endless aging that we saw in Figures 11.1 and 11.2, would people eventually come to fear the long-term consequences of an eternally aging population? Would the share of older people in some countries become so large that the remainder of the population would come to feel a need to enact policies to reduce their influence?

Will Population Aging Ever End? A Regional Perspective

The United Nations expects life expectancy at age 65 to increase in virtually all countries of the world throughout the century. Of course, there is a great deal of uncertainty as to what the speed of increase will be or even if there will be setbacks. We discussed what population aging would look like if life expectancy increases were faster or slower in Chapter 10. As in other chapters, we also take the United Nations forecasts as part of the world that we are exploring. Within that world, things look different depending on which pair of glasses we are wearing, so here we investigate the possibility of a Struldbrug problem using both the conventional *old-age dependency ratio (OADR)* and the *prospective old-age dependency ratio (POADR)*. We published research tangentially related to the Struldbrug problem in Lutz, Sanderson, and Scherbov (2008), when we were studying a different issue, changes in the speed of aging across the world's regions.

The United Nations aggregates countries in various ways. Geographically, it distinguishes six large regions: Africa, Asia, Europe, Latin America and the Caribbean, Northern America, and Oceania. The list of countries in the United Nations' regional aggregates can be found in United Nations (2017d). Figures 11.3a–f present the time paths of the OADR and the POADR for each of the six regions from 2015 to 2100, based on United Nations forecasts.

In Africa, the OADR increases continuously from 2015 through the end of the century. The POADR falls slightly from 2015 to around 2040 and then rises. An increasing number of young adults in Africa keeps the POADR from rising for the next few decades, but eventually the effect of lower predicted fertility there decreases the number of young adults enough that, together with the effect of predicted increases in life expectancy at older ages, it causes the ratio to increase.

In Asia, we see continuous increases in the OADRs. The POADR almost stops growing after 2065. In that year, it is 0.24 and only increases to 0.26 by the end of the century. In Europe, population aging ends around 2065 according to the POADR. The OADR increases during the century, except for a pause between 2060 and 2080. The data for Europe shows that there will be some places that do not see eternal aging. In Latin America and the Caribbean, the OADR increases throughout the century. The POADR also increases, but, between 2080 and 2100, the increase is small. The figures for Northern America provide a particularly striking example of how different measures of population aging affect our perceptions. In Northern America, population aging appears to continue throughout the century, based on the OADR but ends around 2040, when we see things using the POADR. In Oceania, we see continued population aging according to the OADR, but very little increase in the POADR for the last 30 years of the century, where it rises from 0.17 in 2070 to 0.19 in 2100.

When using the POADR, we see the end of population aging very clearly in two of the United Nations major regions, Europe and Northern America. In three of them, Asia, Latin America and the Caribbean, and Oceania, we see very little aging in the last decades of the century. Only in Africa do we see unabated population aging. So, in many places, the end of population aging is already in sight, even though longevity is expected to continue to increase.

The End of Population Aging in Europe

Europe is one of the major regions where the end of population aging is visible using the POADR, but the timing of the end of aging differs

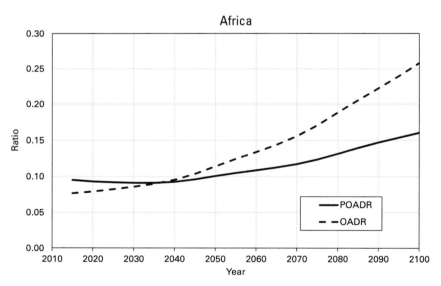

FIGURE 11.3A: Old-age dependency ratio (OADR) and prospective old-age dependency ratio (POADR), Africa.

Data sources: United Nations (2017c); authors' calculations.

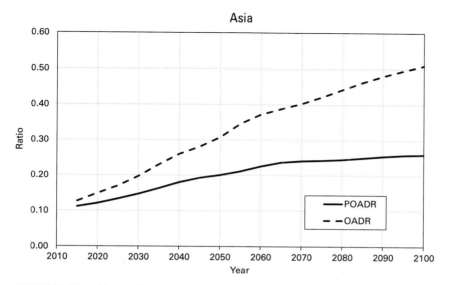

FIGURE 11.3B: Old-age dependency ratio (OADR) and prospective old-age dependency ratio (POADR), Asia.

Data sources: United Nations (2017c); authors' calculations.

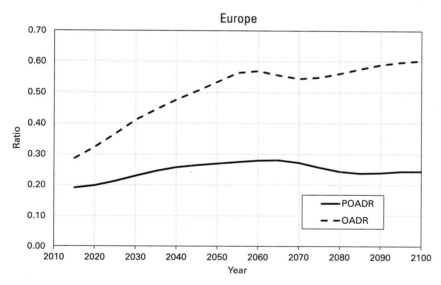

FIGURE 11.3C: Old-age dependency ratio (OADR) and prospective old-age dependency ratio (POADR), Europe.

Data sources: United Nations (2017c); authors' calculations.

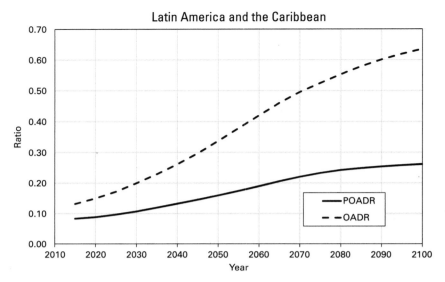

FIGURE 11.3D: Old-age dependency ratio (OADR) and prospective old-age dependency ratio (POADR), Latin America and the Caribbean.

Data sources: United Nations (2017c); authors' calculations.

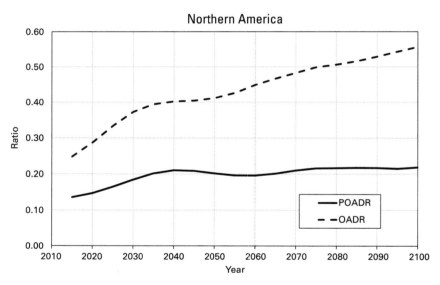

FIGURE 11.3E: Old-age dependency ratio (OADR) and prospective old-age dependency ratio (POADR), Northern America.

Data sources: United Nations (2017c); authors' calculations.

across the continent. In Figure 11.4a–d, we present graphs of the OADR and POADR for the European subregions. In Eastern Europe, waves in the two ratios reflect the population repercussions of the political problems of the 1930s, followed by World War II and then the subsequent recovery. The level of the OADR in 2100 is not far from its peak, which is forecasted to occur in 2060. In contrast, the POADR in 2100 is much lower than its 2060 value, at about the same level as it was in 2030. In Northern and Western Europe, the POADR peaks around 2045 and then declines slowly. Southern Europe shows a different pattern of aging because of its history of rapid fertility decline to persistently low levels. There, the POADR falls only after 2055. In Eastern Europe and Southern Europe, the end of population aging can be seen in both ratios, while in Northern and Western Europe, the OADR increases throughout the century. The details of the timing of the end of population aging depend on historical details, including wars and patterns of fertility change, but almost everywhere in Europe that end is in sight.

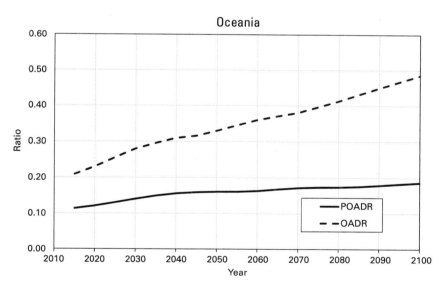

FIGURE 11.3F: Old-age dependency ratio (OADR) and prospective old-age dependency ratio (POADR), Oceania.

Data sources: United Nations (2017c); authors' calculations.

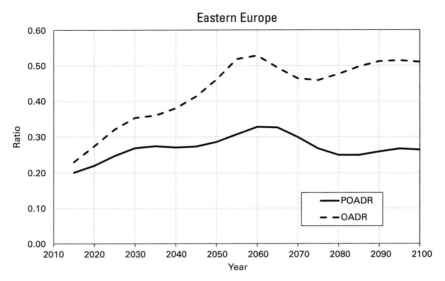

FIGURE 11.4A: Old-age dependency ratio (OADR) and prospective old-age dependency ratio (POADR), Eastern Europe.

Data sources: United Nations (2017c); authors' calculations.

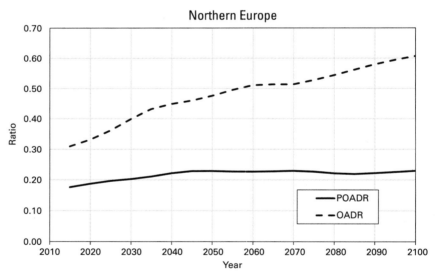

FIGURE 11.4B: Old-age dependency ratio (OADR) and prospective old-age dependency ratio (POADR), Northern Europe.

Data sources: United Nations (2017c); authors' calculations.

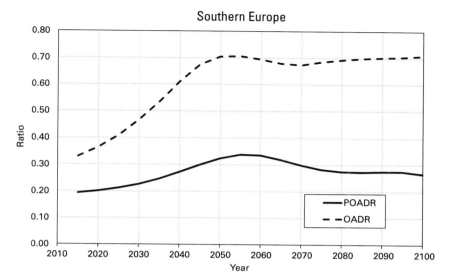

FIGURE 11.4C: Old-age dependency ratio (OADR) and prospective old-age dependency ratio (POADR), Southern Europe.

Data sources: United Nations (2017c); authors' calculations.

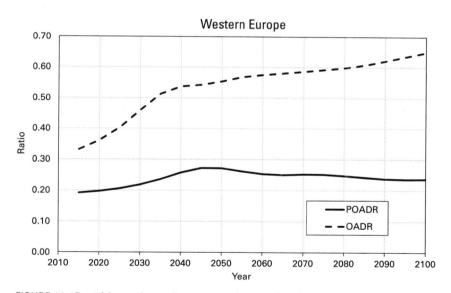

FIGURE 11.4D: Old-age dependency ratio (OADR) and prospective old-age dependency ratio (POADR), Western Europe.

Data sources: United Nations (2017c); authors' calculations.

The End of Population Aging in Some Asian Countries

In Figure 11.5a–e, we investigate the end of population aging in five Asian countries, China, Japan, the Republic of Korea, Thailand, and Iran. Many articles have been written about aging in China. One of them, entitled "China's Aging Population Becoming More of Problem," appeared recently on the website of *Forbes*. According to that article,

> China's getting old. In fact, they are getting older faster than anywhere else in the world. And the Chinese government has a very weak safety net to cover for them all. . . . According to the United Nations, China is ageing more rapidly than almost any country in recent history. China's dependency ratio for retirees could rise as high as 44% by 2050. The dependency ratio compares the difference between those not in the labor force with those who are working, or can work full-time. It is a yardstick geared to measure the pressure on taxable income going to support entitlement programs like Social Security and Medicaid in the U.S. for example. China's aging population is as big a worry as its debt bomb, if not more so, because China can make its debt disappear at the stroke of a pen, but the government cannot make millions of elderly and retirees disappear. (Rapoza 2017)

In Figure 11.5a–e, we can look at the two ratios in selected Asian countries and see how they compare to one another. In China, both ratios rise rapidly from 2015 to 2060. After 2060, the POADR stabilizes, indicating no further population aging. The OADR is roughly constant after 2060 and then continues to climb. The peak of the POADR in China is at a value of 0.35 in 2065. In Japan, the Republic of Korea, Thailand, and Iran, the peaks are similar. They are 0.34 in Japan in 2060; 0.33 in the Republic of Korea in 2060; 0.30 in Thailand in 2060; and 0.35 in Iran in 2065. Even China's OADRs are not particularly high compared with those of the other four countries. From our perspective, the fear of an especially severe aging crisis in China seems overblown. The details of when population aging will end varies with each country's history; nevertheless, population aging is likely to end during this century in all the Asian countries discussed here.

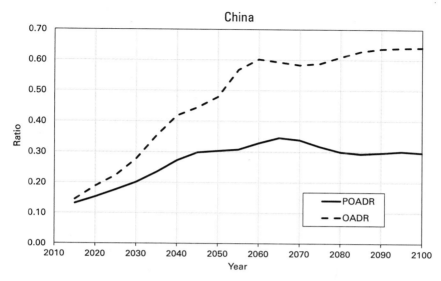

FIGURE 11.5A: Old-age dependency ratio (OADR) and prospective old-age dependency ratio (POADR), China.

Data sources: United Nations (2017c); authors' calculations.

The End of Population Aging in High-Income and Upper-Middle-Income Countries

The United Nations also aggregates countries according to World Bank income categories (World Bank 2017). In Figure 11.6a–d, we show the time paths of the OADRs and the POADRs for people in four groups, those in high-income, middle-income, upper-middle-income, and lower-income countries. In high-income countries, OADR rises rapidly to 2040 and increases more slowly afterward. The POADR rises to 2050 and then remains almost constant. Using that ratio, there would be no additional population aging in high-income countries after the middle of the century.

In middle-income countries, the POADR increases to 2065, when it reaches a level of 0.22 and then increases much more slowly reaching 0.23 in 2100. We would not expect much aging in middle-income countries in the last decades of the century. The World Bank divides middle-income countries into two groups: upper-middle income and

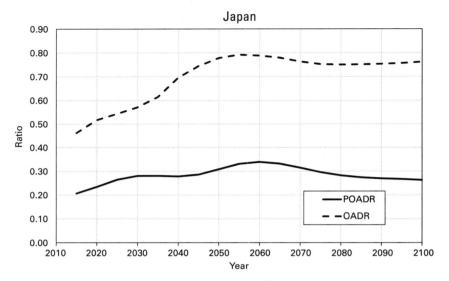

FIGURE 11.5B: Old-age dependency ratio (OADR) and prospective old-age dependency ratio (POADR), Japan.

Data sources: United Nations (2017c); authors' calculations.

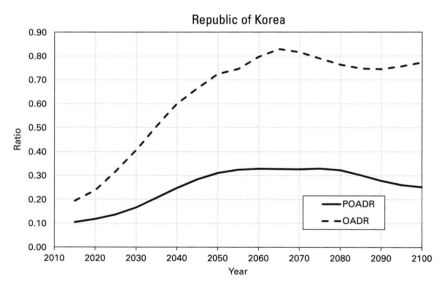

FIGURE 11.5C: Old-age dependency ratio (OADR) and prospective old-age dependency ratio (POADR), Republic of Korea.

Data sources: United Nations (2017c); authors' calculations.

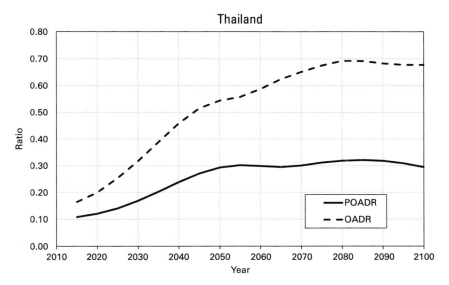

FIGURE 11.5D: Old-age dependency ratio (OADR) and prospective old-age dependency ratio (POADR), Thailand.

Data sources: United Nations (2017c); authors' calculations.

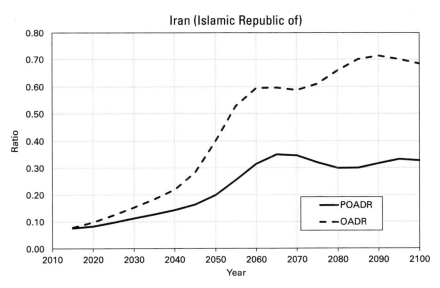

FIGURE 11.5E: Old-age dependency ratio (OADR) and prospective old-age dependency ratio (POADR), Islamic Republic of Iran.

Data sources: United Nations (2017c); authors' calculations.

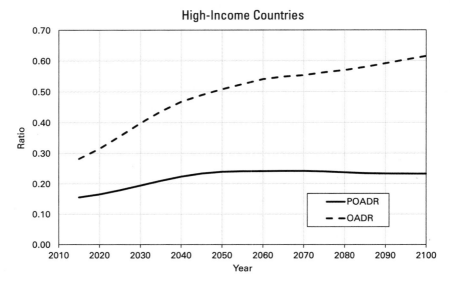

FIGURE 11.6A: Old-age dependency ratio (OADR) and prospective old-age dependency ratio (POADR), high-income countries.

Data sources: United Nations (2017c); authors' calculations.

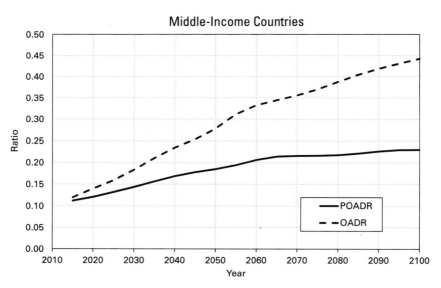

FIGURE 11.6B: Old-age dependency ratio (OADR) and prospective old-age dependency ratio (POADR), middle-income countries.

Data sources: United Nations (2017c); authors' calculations.

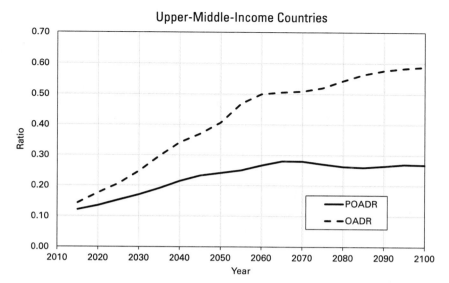

FIGURE 11.6C: Old-age dependency ratio (OADR) and prospective old-age dependency ratio (POADR), upper-middle-income countries.

Data sources: United Nations (2017c); authors' calculations.

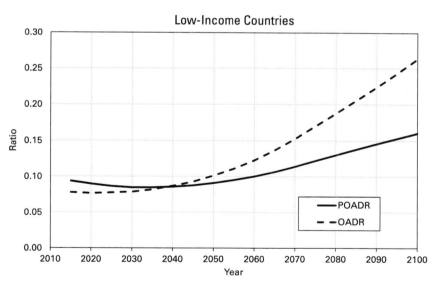

FIGURE 11.6D: Old-age dependency ratio (OADR) and prospective old-age dependency ratio (POADR), low-income countries.

Data sources: United Nations (2017c); authors' calculations.

lower-middle income. We include the graph of the dependency ratios for people in the upper-middle-income countries. There we can see that the POADR is expected to begin declining around 2070. The graphs of the POADR for lower-middle-income countries (not shown here) and for low-income countries do not show a peak in the POADR during this century.

We can see the end of world population aging in some regions and countries by computing our POADRs using United Nations population forecasts. The United Nations recognizes that its forecasts are imprecise because there is considerable uncertainty with regard to the future paths of fertility and mortality. In Sanderson, Scherbov, and Gerland (2017), we produced probabilistic POADRs using the United Nations' probabilistic population and life table forecasts and demonstrated that, taking demographic uncertainties into account, the end of population aging is still observed with roughly the same timing as in the figures above. We provide more details about the probabilistic forecasts in the appendix to this chapter.

Conclusion

The end of population aging is not something that is hypothetical. It is built into current age structures. Massive increases in migration could postpone the end of population aging in some countries, but even with the increased migration flows that have been currently observed, the postponement would generally be very modest.

We need to be cautious about analyses of population aging that begin with pictures of 65-year-olds living in a poor rural area of a country, accompanied by a warning to the reader that there would be many more people like them in the future. Tomorrow's 65-year-olds are not likely to be like today's 65-year-olds. They will be richer, more educated, more likely to live in urban areas, and likely will have experienced a life of better nutrition and healthcare.

The end of population aging in the future, when computed using our new measures, does not mean the end of concern about changes in age structures now. Population aging will still be challenging. If public policies continue to be formulated on the basis of fixed chronological ages, a modern version of the Struldbrug problem may yet arise.

II

Appendix

In Chapter 11, we discussed the end of population aging. The demographic future is uncertain, so, in this appendix, we address the issue of how certain we are that population aging will come to an end in some parts of the world during this century, even though life expectancies continue to increase. In Sanderson, Scherbov, and Gerland (2017), we combined two demographic methodologies, the United Nations' probabilistic population forecasts and our *prospective* measures of population aging. The United Nations uses its database of historical estimates and a forecasting methodology called Bayesian hierarchical modeling (Raftery et al. 2012) to produce thousands of possible future paths of fertility and mortality, which are then combined with existing population age structures to produce probabilistic population forecasts.

We apply conventional measures of aging and our prospective ones to those probabilistic forecasts and observe the differences. We present these in Figures 11.A1 through 11.A4, which are for China, Germany, Iran, and the United States. Each of the figures is composed of six graphs. On the left-hand side, we show the probabilistic forecasts of three conventional measures of population aging: (1) the *proportion of the population categorized as being old (PO)*, (2) the *old-age dependency ratio (OADR)*, and (3) *the median age (MA)* of the population. Next to them on the right-hand side, we show their prospective counterparts: (1) the *prospective proportion of the population who are considered old (PPO)*, (2) the *prospective old-age dependency ratio (POADR)*, and (3) the *prospective median age (PMA)*.

Using all three prospective probabilistic measures, we can see that population aging is highly likely to end before the end of the century in China, Germany, and the United States. This is less clear in Iran where a rapid fall in fertility in the past has led to an age structure with large variations in the sizes of cohorts. In Figure 11.5a, we presented the deterministic forecasts of the OADR and POADR for China, and,

Probability Distributions of Conventional and Prospective Measures of Aging

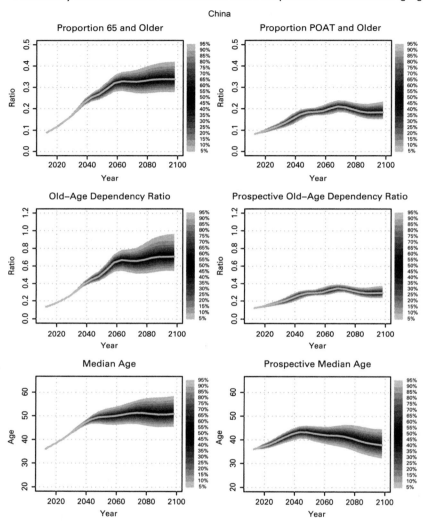

FIGURE 11.A1: Probabilistic forecasts of three conventional and probabilistic measures of population aging, China, 2013–2098.

Source: Sanderson, Scherbov, and Gerland (2017, figure 2).

Probability Distributions of Conventional and Prospective Measures of Aging

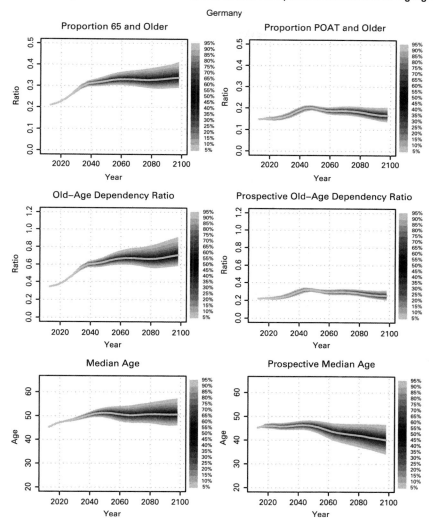

FIGURE 11.A2: Probabilistic forecasts of three conventional and probabilistic measures of population aging, Germany, 2013–2098.

Source: Sanderson, Scherbov, and Gerland (2017, figure 3).

Probability Distributions of Conventional and Prospective Measures of Aging

Iran (Islamic Republic of)

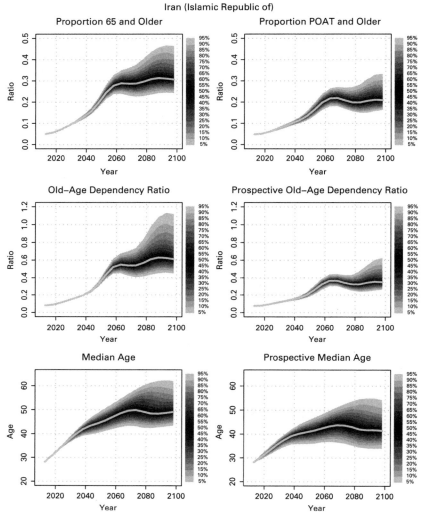

FIGURE 11.A3: Probabilistic forecasts of three conventional and probabilistic measures of population aging, Islamic Republic of Iran, 2013–2098.

Source: Sanderson, Scherbov, and Gerland (2017, figure 4).

Probability Distributions of Conventional and Prospective Measures of Aging

United States

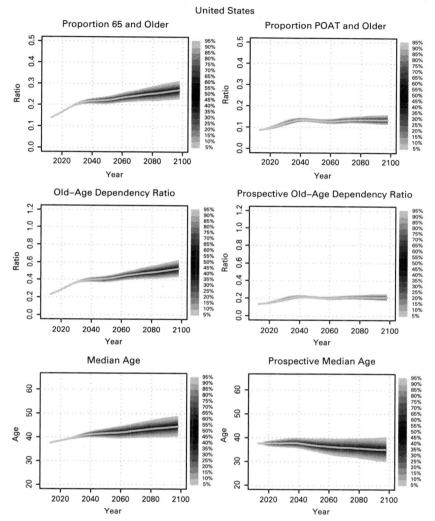

FIGURE 11.A4: Probabilistic forecasts of three conventional and probabilistic measures of population aging, United States, 2013–2098.

Source: Sanderson, Scherbov, and Gerland (2017, figure 5).

in Figure 11.5e, the deterministic forecasts of those ratios for Iran. As can be seen in Figure 11.A1, the uncertainty of the forecasted POADR in China is small, as can be seen by the narrowness of the shaded area. The end of population aging that we saw in Figure 11.5a can also be seen in Figure 11.A1. In Iran, the forecast is much more uncertain. The POADR may begin to decrease during this century or continue to increase. The United Nations' probabilistic forecasts do not allow a more definitive statement.

12

Intergenerationally Equitable Normal Pension Ages

ONE OF THE most pressing problems with respect to population has to do with national pension finance. In March 2017, we searched Google for the phrase "pension crisis" and the result was that there were "about 260,000" web pages in English. Out of those roughly 260,000 web pages, around two-tenths of 1 percent of them included the phrase "pension crisis solved." However, the phrase "pension crisis" does not fully reflect the height of people's concerns. The phrase "pension tsunami" was found in around 431,000 web pages.

When we looked into the causes of these reported crises and tsunamis, there were, of course, the usual statements about politicians and their promises. Aside from these, the main explanations of the crises were unanticipated demographic changes or, perhaps more accurately, demographic changes that were unanticipated by policymakers. When demographic changes are slow, predictions tend to be good because tomorrow's changes will be much like yesterday's changes. When those changes are faster, they can cause, and now have caused, surprises. Inevitably, basing pension systems on long-term demographic forecasts will sometimes result in sustainability and, sometimes, crises. Blaming pension crises on unanticipated demographic changes is a bit like blaming death through Russian roulette on unanticipated bullet placement.

We traveled to Stockholm, where we drank aquavit with friends. We are about to propose a toast to the Swedish national pension system. It is a system that flexibly incorporates changing life expectancy and, with that, eliminates pension crises. The pension system that we describe in this chapter is similar to the one currently implemented there. The Swedish experience demonstrates that it is possible to take the changing characteristics of people into account in designing public policies (OECD 2015).

Normal Public Pension Ages Are Changing

The first nationwide public pension system passed the German parliament in 1889. The 1889 pension was first broached to the German parliament in a letter sent to it by the Emperor William I at the urging of then Chancellor Otto von Bismarck. The Emperor's letter included a passage that is translated as "those that are disabled from work by age and invalidity have a well-grounded claim to care from the state" (Social Security, n.d.). Before that time, there were pension plans for specific groups, particularly soldiers. Bismarck's pension system had several revolutionary features. Most importantly, its applicability was not conditioned on specific acts of service to the state. Thus, for the first time, receiving a state pension became a right. The pension age was initially set at 70. We do not know what life expectancy was in Bismarck's Germany in 1889, but we do know it for some surrounding countries. In Belgium, the life expectancy of 70-year-old men in 1889 was 8.3 years. In Denmark, it was 9.1 years. It was 8.3 years, 8.6 years, and 7.5 years in France, the Netherlands, and Switzerland, respectively (University of California, Berkeley, and Max Planck Institute for Demographic Research 2017). So, a plausible guess is that, in 1889, the life expectancy of a 70-year-old man in Germany was around 8 years. If Bismarck's pension plan had been written in terms of a remaining life expectancy instead of a chronological age, the pension age for men in Germany today would be around 80.

Normal public pension ages are in the process of changing in many countries. An important source of information on public pension systems is the OECD publication *Pensions at a Glance* (OECD 2015). There we find this description of some of these changes:

> The last decade has been a period of intense reform activity in the area of pensions. . . . The most visible progress has been made in

raising official pension ages. Many countries have been moving this key parameter beyond the mark of 65 years. As highlighted in previous editions of Pensions at a Glance, 67 *has indeed become the new 65*, and several countries are going even further towards ages closer to 70. (OECD 2015, 9, 23, 25; emphasis added)

Indeed, in national pensions systems in OECD countries 67 has become the new 65. But in our view, having a fixed normal pension age of 67 is little better than having a fixed age of 65. How many years would it be until people are told that in terms of pension age 70 is the new 67? What is needed is a new view of pension ages, one that takes the changing characteristics of people into account. It is not an impossible task. Sweden and other countries have devised a way to do just that (Sanderson and Scherbov 2015a).

Demographically Indexed Public Policies: The Work of Shoven and Goda

In Bismarck's time it would have been impossible to consider a pension plan based on longevity because the necessary statistical information was not available. Nowadays, however, in many countries the requisite data are available. Shoven and Goda (2010) performed an interesting thought experiment that is relevant to this discussion. They studied the difference it would make if public policies in the United States were written using chronological age or using some dynamically changing demographic variable, such as remaining life expectancy. They studied seven different policies based on chronological age. We focus here on their results regarding the age at which people could obtain a full public pension (social security pension).

Pension policies are often written into law using chronological ages, but they could also be written in terms of some characteristics, such as remaining life expectancy or 1-year mortality rate, among others. In the terminology in this book, chronological ages where the level of some characteristic is held constant are called *constant characteristic ages*. In general, the problem with developing policies based on constant characteristic ages is that there are different constant characteristic ages depending on the characteristic used. Using our terminology, we would say that Shoven and Goda (2010) computed constant characteristic ages based on four life table-based characteristics: remaining life expectancy, 1-year mortality rate, a constant percentage of life expectancy at birth, and a constant percentage of the expected total lifetimes of people who survive to age 20 (remaining life expectancy at age 20 plus 20 years). Shoven and Goda (2010) call their ages "inflation-adjusted ages." We present their results in Table 12.1.

In the top panel of the table, Shoven and Goda provide constant characteristic ages in 2004 where the level of the characteristic is fixed at two different levels. The first is that of people of age 65 in 1935. The legislation in the United States, which established a national pension system, was passed in 1935 and set the normal pension age at 65. The second is age 67 in 1983. The reform of the US pension system in 1983 raised the normal pension age to 67 for people born in 1960 and later. The bottom panel of the table gives constant characteristic ages in 2050 for the levels of characteristics observed in 2004 at age 65 and at age 67.

Table 12.1 shows that, if the Social Security Act had set the full pension age at the remaining life expectancy at age 65 in 1935, the full pension age for men in 2004 would have been between 73 and 74 years old and between 71 and 72 years old for women. If, instead of writing the legislation in terms of life expectancy, it had been written in terms of annual survival rates, the full pension ages in 2004 would have been even higher.

By taking the important step of showing how a variety of US policies would be different depending on whether they were written in terms of chronological age or some relevant demographic criterion, Shoven and Goda (2010) also uncovered an important problem. There are a number of demographic characteristics that can be used in policy formation. There needs to be a rationale for using a particular one in a particular context. Otherwise, the demographic indexation of ages in public policies could lead to endless political bickering.

A Principle for Determining Normal Pension Ages: Intergenerational Equity

It certainly matters how pension ages are determined, but, currently, there are no general rules for doing this. Instead of determining the

Table 12.1 Constant characteristic ages based on four characteristics

Level of characteristic observed at . . .	Constant characteristic ages in 2004			
	Age 65 in 1935		Age 67 in 1983	
	Men	Women	Men	Women
Characteristic				
Remaining life expectancy	73	71	69	67
1-year mortality rate	75	73	71	68
Percentage of life expectancy at birth	83	81.9	70.6	68.3
Percentage of life expectancy conditional on reaching age 20	76.1	74.8	70	67.9

Level of characteristic observed at . . .	Constant characteristic ages in 2050			
	Age 65 in 2004		Age 67 in 2004	
	Men	Women	Men	Women
Characteristic				
Remaining life expectancy	68	67	70	69
1-year mortality rate	69	68	71	70
Percentage of life expectancy at birth	69.2	67.9	71.3	70
Percentage of life expectancy conditional on reaching age 20	68.7	67.5	70.9	69.6

Data source: Shoven and Goda (2010, 152, table 4.1; 154, table 4.2).
Note: Life expectancy conditional of reaching age 20 is the remaining life expectancy at age 20 plus 20 years. Shoven and Goda rounded the constant characteristic ages obtained using remaining life expectancy and the 1-year survival rate downward to the nearest integer.

normal pension age based on some principles, the argument is often made that pension arrangements must be changed because they are too expensive to maintain. The solution proposed is to provide pensioners with less money. However, this argument is conceptually flawed. If the pension policy itself is appropriate, then the question of how to fund pensions requires more general consideration. Perhaps increased pension expenditure could be funded by some combination of decreasing subsidies to favored sectors of the economy and increasing taxes on polluting activities. After all, we do not hear the argument that because healthcare for children has grown more expensive, they should be provided with fewer inoculations. If pension arrangements are to be changed, there should be a clear justification for doing so. Without such a justification, pension ages tend to be changed episodically and under financial duress. This is not the best approach to policymaking. In democratic countries with aging populations, without an accepted rationale for setting pension policy, it might become progressively more difficult to raise pension ages, resulting in policies which favor older generations at the expense of younger ones.

An important element in current problems with pension sustainability is that full pension ages have often been legislated years in advance. In the United States, for example, changes in full pension ages planned between 2021 and 2027 were written into law in 1983. Since current problems with pension sustainability are occurring because of unanticipated demographic changes, it may well be wise not to repeat the procedure of producing pension arrangements based on new anticipated demographic changes, which easily could go as much awry as the previous set of incorrectly anticipated changes.

In this chapter, we propose a general principle for setting normal pension ages, intergenerational equity. Normal pension ages based on intergenerational equity have the advantages of clarity, consistency, and sustainability. Many current pension systems are not intergenerationally equitable. If full pension ages and the full pension payout rates are fixed, then successive generations, each of which lives more years after the full pension age, receive more and more pension income over their lifetimes. This additional income must be paid by younger generations. Such an arrangement is not intergenerationally equitable because some generations fare better than others.

It is impossible for us to discuss the setting of intergenerationally equitable pension ages in individual countries in full detail. Pension systems are too complex and our knowledge of their details too scanty. Instead, we explain it in the context of a model of a highly simplified pension system. The maxim that "all models are wrong, but some are useful" applies here as well. The simplification allows us to see things that we otherwise could not see and answer questions that we otherwise could not answer. But these come at the cost of ignoring the details.

The highly simplified equitable pension system that we have in mind is based on two principles.

Principle 1: A group of people entering the pension system at age 20 would receive back in pension what they paid in. No money would be taken from any cohort to fund the pensions of any other cohort.

Principle 2: The pension payment that people in each generation get is the same proportion of their incomes after their pension taxes. No generation will be favored by a particularly large pension payout compared to what they and others are paying in.

These two principles encapsulate a particular view of intergenerational fairness. It assumes that there are no subsidies from one generation to another. There are, however, situations where subsidies might be appropriate. For example, one generation may have lived through a war and society might find it equitable to subsidize those people. In the short term, there may be good reasons for one generation to subsidize another, but in our simplified pension system there cannot be ever-increasing transfers from the young to the old or from the old to the young.

The very simple model of an intergenerationally equitable pension age is not designed to approximate pension ages in individual countries. Its purpose is to demonstrate understandable principles that can be easily communicated to people. The intergenerationally equitable normal pension age has several uses. First, it can be used to assess whether the normal pension age in a country is increasing faster or slower than the intergenerationally equitable one. Second, it can be used in cross-country comparisons, because it is computed on a consistent basis for all countries (Sanderson and Scherbov 2015a). Intergenerationally equitable pension ages can also be used to compute a new sort of dependency ratio. In the numerator, we could put all the people who are at or above the intergenerationally equitable pension age and put all the people from age 20 to the intergenerationally equitable pension age in the denominator. Roughly speaking, this is the ratio of all the people eligible to receive a pension to all those who could be contributing to the pension system. We have computed this ratio in Sanderson and Scherbov (2015b) and shown that it increases less rapidly than the conventional *old-age dependency ratio.*

Model-Based Intergenerationally Equitable Pension Ages

In the appendix to this chapter, we write the equations that correspond to the two principles above. They show that intergenerationally equitable normal pension ages are things that we are now able to see with our new glasses. To be precise, those pension ages are constant characteristic ages based on the *life course ratio.* In other words, intergenerationally equitable normal pension ages are the chronological ages that keep the fraction of adult lifetimes in which people are eligible for a normal pension fixed.

We provide an example showing how intergenerationally equitable normal pension ages are computed in Table 12.2. The level of the life course ratio that produces intergenerationally equitable normal pension ages depends on the pension tax rate, which is the fraction of income that is paid into the pension system each year, and the replacement ratio, which is the ratio of annual pension receipts to average annual income after pension taxes. These two numbers determine a fixed value of the life course ratio. As a practical matter, we do not know these numbers for most countries, so we take a shortcut and start with a predetermined value of the life course ratio. In Table 12.2, we start with the level of the life course ratio observed for 65-year-old German women in 2013. The value of their life course ratio was 0.3, indicating that 30 percent of all the person-years that would be lived by German women after age 20 would also be lived at age 65 and beyond, given the survival rates of 2013. We show this in columns 1 and 2 of Table 12.2.

Given a life course ratio of 0.3, we can find the ages in other years when German women would have the same life course ratio. Using projected life tables, we see that German 65.82-year-old women in 2020 would have that value of the life course ratio (column 3) as would 67.09-year-old women in 2030 (column 4), 68.34-year-old women in 2040 (column 5), and 69.62-year-old women in 2050 (column 6). All the ages in Table 12.2 are consistent, intergenerationally equitable normal pension ages. If 65 was the intergenerationally equitable pension age in 2013, then the intergenerationally equitable normal pension age in 2050 would be 69.62.

Table 12.2 Example of the determination of intergenerationally equitable normal pension ages for German women

(1)	(2)	(3)	(4)	(5)	(6)
Life course ratio for 65-year-old women in 2013	Age at life course ratio=0.30 in 2013	Age at life course ratio=0.30 in 2020	Age at life course ratio=0.30 in 2030	Age at life course ratio=0.30 in 2040	Age at life course ratio=0.30 in 2050
0.30	65	65.82	67.09	68.34	69.62

Data sources: University of California, Berkeley, and Max Planck Institute for Demographic Research (2017); authors' calculations.

We show intergenerationally equitable pension ages in Tables 12.3a and 12.3b for selected countries from 2013 to 2050 using data from the European Demographic Datasheet 2014 (VID and IIASA 2014). The table is constructed by fixing the life course ratio at the level observed in the country for people 65 years old in 2013; therefore, the figures for German women are the same as those in Table 12.2.

The figures in Tables 12.3a and 12.3b are quite close to some already legislated changes. For example, in France, the normal pension age is planned to increase to 67 in 2023, in Germany to 67 in 2029, and to 67 in the United Kingdom in 2028 (OECD 2013, 2015). While increases in intergenerationally equitable pension ages are not designed to predict increases in national pension ages that are already enacted, the consistency of those changes shows that constant characteristic ages

Table 12.3a Intergenerationally equitable normal pension ages for women in selected European countries, 2013, 2020, 2030, 2040, and 2050

Women, 2013 = 65	2013	2020	2030	2040	2050	Months per year
Country						
Bulgaria	65.00	65.42	66.63	67.83	69.13	1.3
Czech Republic	65.00	66.00	67.49	69.00	70.41	1.8
France	65.00	65.65	66.88	68.03	69.28	1.4
Georgia	65.00	65.37	66.55	67.77	69.04	1.3
Germany	65.00	65.82	67.09	68.34	69.62	1.5
Greece	65.00	65.97	67.32	68.59	69.88	1.6
Ireland	65.00	65.68	66.86	68.07	69.31	1.4
Italy	65.00	65.65	66.89	68.13	69.37	1.4
Latvia	65.00	65.68	66.88	68.13	69.36	1.4
Russian Federation	65.00	65.37	66.46	67.50	68.58	1.2
Serbia	65.00	65.63	66.90	68.18	69.49	1.5
Slovakia	65.00	65.78	67.04	68.30	69.61	1.5
Spain	65.00	65.41	66.63	67.85	69.09	1.3
Sweden	65.00	65.70	66.90	68.14	69.40	1.4
United Kingdom	65.00	65.68	66.97	68.19	69.41	1.4
Average						1.4

Source: Sanderson and Scherbov (2015a, 204, table 4a).

Note: The life course ratio is fixed at the level observed in the country for 65-year-olds in 2013. Months per year is the average number of months per year that the intergenerationally equitable pension age changes between 2013 and 2050.

Table 12.3b   Intergenerationally equitable normal pension ages for men
in selected European countries, 2013, 2020, 2030, 2040,
and 2050

Men, 2013 = 65	2013	2020	2030	2040	2050	Months per year
Country						
Bulgaria	65.00	65.60	66.96	68.31	69.69	1.5
Czech Republic	65.00	65.99	67.58	69.16	70.61	1.8
France	65.00	66.09	67.52	68.74	70.02	1.6
Georgia	65.00	66.17	67.54	68.89	70.27	1.7
Germany	65.00	66.00	67.45	68.70	69.99	1.6
Greece	65.00	66.19	67.58	68.84	70.15	1.7
Ireland	65.00	65.56	66.71	67.89	69.10	1.3
Italy	65.00	65.57	66.84	68.14	69.40	1.4
Latvia	65.00	66.17	67.80	69.39	70.83	1.9
Russian Federation	65.00	65.69	67.33	68.81	70.22	1.7
Serbia	65.00	65.97	67.27	68.54	69.85	1.6
Slovakia	65.00	65.92	67.46	68.85	70.26	1.7
Spain	65.00	65.61	67.05	68.35	69.64	1.5
Sweden	65.00	65.66	66.87	68.07	69.34	1.4
United Kingdom	65.00	65.58	66.82	68.00	69.23	1.4
Average						1.6

Source: Sanderson and Scherbov (2015a, 205, table 5b).
Note: The life course ratio is fixed at the level observed in the country for
65-year-olds in 2013. Months per year is the average number of months per year that
the intergenerationally equitable pension age changes between 2013 and 2050.

can also be helpful in interpreting what we see here. An interesting
observation from Tables 12.3a and 12.3b concerns Ireland. The economic crisis in 2008–2009 led Ireland to raise the normal pension age
to 68 in 2028. In the table, the intergenerationally equitable normal
pension age would be 66.86 in 2030 for women and 66.71 for men. This
suggests that economic problems may have led Ireland to raise the
normal pension age faster than would be intergenerationally equitable.

Conclusion

Perhaps the most important advantage of our intergenerationally equitable normal pension age is that it is a pension age based on easily
understandable and widely accepted principles. It is not meant to be a

simplification of the process of setting normal pension ages on a country by country basis. Instead, it answers the question of how an intergenerationally equitable pension age should change as demographic conditions change. Instead of lurching from one pension reform to another when there are fiscal problems, the intergenerationally equitable normal pension age could be used to help make changes more predictable and more equitable. Without an accepted rationale for changing the normal pension age as life expectancy increases, there is a danger that pension age changes could make pension systems less equitable. In a democratic country with an aging population, politicians looking for votes could countenance pension systems that become more favorable to the elderly and less favorable to the young. We discussed this problem in Sanderson and Scherbov (2007).

A desirable feature of an intergenerationally equitable pension system is that it should not increase intragenerational inequality over time. Populations may have disadvantaged groups that have below-average incomes and above-average mortality rates. Pension systems alone cannot solve problems related to income inequality. A wide variety of other public policies are needed to address this, but pension systems can help. In practice, pension systems deal with such disadvantaged groups in two ways. First, the schedule that relates pension contributions to pension payouts can be progressive, in the sense that the ratio of payouts to contributions is lower for richer people than for poorer people. This is the case in the United States and many other countries (OECD 2015). The second is the provision of a noncontributory pension. This is found in Canada, the Czech Republic, Estonia, Ireland, and New Zealand, for example (OECD 2015). In the appendix, we discuss the relationship between intergenerational and intragenerational equity more formally.

Life expectancies are generally increasing, and countries have choices about how to adjust their pension systems. One choice is to ignore the life expectancy increase. If a pension crisis ensues, the country could make an abrupt change and the current generation of politicians could blame demographic changes that were not anticipated by the prior generation of politicians. The alternative is to engage in a social discussion of the rationale upon which the country's pension system should be based. If it is to be based on intergenerational equity, then the sort of ideas that we have been discussing throughout this book can help.

We must add an important word of caution here. If we were to ask economists what the level of prices will be in, say, Azerbaijan half a century from now, they are likely to tell us that no economist could answer that question with a reasonable degree of accuracy. But if we were to ask demographers what life expectancy at, say, age 65 would be in Azerbaijan half a century from now, they might point us to the United Nations' website where the answer, at this writing, is that in 2070–2075, the remaining life expectancy of Azerbaijani women at age 65 is forecasted to be 20.08 years and is forecasted to be 16.54 years for men (United Nations 2017c, 2017e). Long-term forecasts of life expectancy will almost certainly be more accurate than long-term forecasts of price levels. Nevertheless, there is still considerable uncertainty about what a country's life table will look like half a century from now. Unforeseen changes in mortality patterns are inevitable and pension systems need to be flexible enough to take such changes into account.

In the old days, when people were wearing eyeglasses that were designed a century ago, they were blind to the changing characteristics of people. All 65-year-olds, for example, were assumed to be like other 65-year-olds in every place in the world and forever. In the realm of public pensions, countries were forced to see things differently and as the OECD wrote: "67 has indeed become the new 65." Nevertheless, few countries have put on glasses that allow them to see that the changing characteristics of people is an ongoing process. Without this understanding, there are likely to be more pension problems. It need not come as a surprise to us that one day 70 will become the new 67. With the proper glasses, we can see this coming and act appropriately.

Mathematical Appendix

The highly simplified equitable pension system that we have in mind is based on two principles.

Principle 1: A group of people entering the pension system at age 20 would receive back in pension what they paid in. No money will be taken from any cohort to fund the pensions of any other cohort.

Principle 2: The pension payment that people in each generation receive is the same proportion of their incomes after their pension taxes. No generation will be favored by a particularly large pension payout compared to what they and others are paying in.

We express the first principle using the formula,

$$(T_{20,i,g} - T_{p,i,g}) \cdot y_{i,g} \cdot t_i = T_{p,i,g} \cdot \pi_{i,g}. \tag{12.A1}$$

$T_{a,i,g}$ is the number of *person-years* lived from age a onward. As an example of person-years, consider a population with two people in it. Starting at age 20, person 1 lives 50.3 more years and person 2 lives 60.7 more years. The total of the person-years lived by the two of them is 50.3 plus 60.7 or 111. In equation (12.A1), p is the *intergenerationally equitable normal pension age*, i refers to a country, g refers to a generation, $y_{i,g}$ is the average income of people in country i and generation g subject to the pension tax. t_i is the pension tax rate in country i, and $\pi_{i,g}$ is the pension amount received by people of generation g in country i.

The second principle is expressed in the equation,

$$\pi_{i,g} = \beta_i \cdot (1 - t_i) \cdot y_{i,g}. \tag{12.A2}$$

β_i is the ratio of the pension payout for people of generation g in country i to the average income of people in that generation after paying the pension tax. In other words, β_i is the replacement ratio in country i. Note that the pension tax rate and the replacement rate are assumed to be the same for each generation.

Substituting the value of $\pi_{i,g}$ from equation (12.A2) into equation (12. A1) yields,

$$\frac{T_{p,i,g}}{T_{20,i,g}} = \frac{t_i}{\beta_i \cdot (1 - t_i) + t_i}. \qquad (12.A3)$$

The ratio on the left-hand side of the equation is just the *life course ratio* that we discussed in Chapter 6. What is on the right-hand side of the equation depends only on the country and does not change over time or with the level of income, so equation (12.A3) determines p, the intergenerationally equitable pension age. The intergenerationally equitable pension age is also a constant characteristic age, because the level of the characteristic, $T_{p,i,g} / T_{20,i,g}$, is fixed once β_i and t_i, two country-specific constants, are known.

For many countries, however, we do not have information on the pension tax rate and the replacement ratio. Instead of starting with an observed value of the right-hand side of equation (12.A3), we can choose the life course schedule from a particular year and an age. From these two, we could read off the corresponding value of the life course ratio. Holding that value constant allows us to compute the *constant characteristic ages* in other years. These ages provide us with a time series of intergenerationally equitable pension ages consistent with the original choice of age and year.

So far, we have dealt with the case of cohorts that were homogeneous in life expectancy. An important issue arises when we allow the possibility that cohorts are not homogeneous in life expectancy and there is a disadvantaged subgroup with a lower life expectancy. To analyze this case, we return to equation (12.A3). A rearrangement of that equation expresses the replacement ratio in terms of the pension tax rate and demographic factors:

$$\beta_i = \left[\left(\frac{T_{20,i,g}}{T_{p,i,g}} - 1 \right) \right] \cdot \frac{t_i}{1 - t_i}. \qquad (12.A4)$$

β_i is the value of the replacement ratio which would result in the cohort receiving as much in pension payouts as it put in. If a disadvantaged subgroup of generation g were to receive as much in pension payouts as it put in and its pension age is the same as in equation (12. A3), its replacement ratio would be,

$$\beta_{t_i}^d = \left[\left(\frac{T_{20,i,g}^d}{T_{p,i,g}^d} - 1 \right) \right] \cdot \frac{t_i}{1 - t_i}, \qquad (12.A5)$$

where the superscript d refers to the disadvantaged subgroup. For the subgroup to be disadvantaged it must be that $\frac{T_{20,i,g}^d}{T_{p,i,g}^d} > \frac{T_{20,i,g}}{T_{p,i,g}}$ or, in other words, that people in the disadvantaged population get fewer years in the pension ages compared to the years they spend in the contributing ages. Therefore, the replacement ratio should be greater for those in the disadvantaged group.

The proportional increase in replacement ratio, β, that the disadvantaged cohort should get relative to the others is

$$\frac{\beta_i^d}{\beta_i} = \frac{\left[\left(\dfrac{T_{20,i,g}^d}{T_{p,i,g}^d} - 1 \right) \right]}{\left[\left(\dfrac{T_{20,i,g}}{T_{p,i,g}} - 1 \right) \right]}. \qquad (12.A6)$$

The ratio of the replacement rate for the disadvantaged compared to the rest of the population depends only on the survival rate differences between the two populations and is independent of the level of income of the two populations and the level of the pension tax. Equation (12.A6) provides information that can be used in developing progressive replacement rate schedules.

It is difficult and politically contentious to decide which groups to favor with higher replacement rates. Heroin addicts generally have shorter live expectancies than people who are not addicted. Certainly, this could not be a reason to reward those addicts with higher pensions. It would be possible to provide people with less education with higher replacement rates, but this would provide an incentive for people to obtain less education. As a practical matter, pension plans deal with subgroup differences in mortality rates through the correlation between income and longevity. The replacement rates of people with lower incomes are often higher than those with higher incomes. This is accomplished through replacement rate schedules that are progressive and through the provision of noncontributory pensions. Progressive replacement rate schedules, a noncontributory pension in addition to a contributory one, or both are found in most of the pension systems of high-income OECD countries.

Within the highly simplified framework we use here, even though the disadvantaged group has a higher replacement ratio, there is no subsidy to it from other groups. The disadvantaged group also gets back what it pays in but no more. The higher replacement rate is the result of two factors. First, a smaller percentage of the disadvantaged group survives to the pension age and, second, those who do survive live on average fewer years than people who are not disadvantaged.

The highly simplified model presented here does not explicitly deal with baby-boom and baby-bust generations, but it's easy enough to see what it would imply for them. In that model, every generation finances its own pensions. A baby-boom cohort would pay into the pension system more than the system pays out to the comparatively smaller cohorts receiving a pension. A fund would be built up while the baby boomers were working and would eventually be used up to pay their pensions later. In the long term, because each generation funds its own pensions, there are no pension crises.

The model can also be used to help us understand why pension crises exist. Equation (12.A3) shows that in an intergenerationally equitable pension system three parameters of the pension system, the full pension age, the pension tax rate, and the replacement ratio are interrelated. If we know two of them, they determine the third. However, policymakers are not always aware of this and set the three in a way that is inconsistent with intergenerational equity and sustainability. Sometimes this results in the pension crises that we observe.

There is no financial discounting in the model. Financial discounting is controversial. No one knows exactly what discount rate to use or whether the discount rate is the same for younger and older people. Incorporating financial discounting would enormously complicate equations (12.A1) and (12.A2) and, in the end, provide little additional insight. There is, however, a form of demographic discounting in the model. People at the intergenerationally equitable full pension age receive more over their lifetime than they paid in.

Not everyone participating in the pension system survives to the full pension age. Since in the model each generation finances its own pensions, the money paid into the pension system by those who die before the full pension age gets redistributed to those who survive. This additional payment is compensation for bearing the risk of dying before the full pension age.

Many pension systems allow people to choose when to begin receiving their pensions within a specified age range. The model provides a perspective on how pension payouts should be computed for people who choose to begin their pensions at different ages. Equation (12.A4) shows the relationship between the replacement ratio and the ratio, T_{20}/T_p, where T_p is the number of person-years lived from the age at which people choose to start their pension to the end of their lives. When people can choose when to start their pension, equation (12.A4) gives the intergenerationally equitable replacement ratio for the chosen age.

13

Choosing Which Pair of Glasses to Wear

WE HAVE NOW TRAVELED to New York City, the home of the United Nations Population Division. When people discuss almost any topic related to population aging, they usually rely on the United Nations' data. The meticulous work that goes into producing those data is often underappreciated because they are so easily available on the United Nations' website. Although the Population Division deserves more praise for its technical prowess and statistical analysis, we are here for a different purpose. We are here because of an interesting problem that the Population Division has now inadvertently created for demographers and others interested in population aging.

The World Health Organization supports our argument that aging should not be conceptualized on the basis of fixed chronological ages but rather be based on the characteristics of people (WHO 2015). There can be no denying that those characteristics, such as remaining life expectancy, differ from place to place and over time. The problem arises because the United Nations now gives people a choice between two old-age dependency ratios, one that uses a fixed chronological age as its old-age threshold, the conventional *old-age dependency ratio (OADR)* and one where the old-age threshold reflects changing life expectancies, the *prospective old-age dependency ratio (POADR)*. In discussing population aging, people now have a problem. They have to choose one or the other, because the implications for understanding population aging and formulating appropriate policies on the basis of each of them are so different.

The Necessity of Choice

For over a decade, we have been writing about population aging from a new perspective, one that takes the characteristics of people into account. In 2017, the United Nations accepted one of our measures, the POADR. This measure of population aging now appears along with the older measures in *World Population Ageing 2017* (United Nations 2017a, 2017f). As a result, people interested in population aging have a choice of measures. However, this choice is associated with a problem. When demographers discuss population aging, are they going to say things like "on the one hand, using the POADR, we can see that population aging is likely to come to an end in Western Europe during this century and, on the other hand, that, using the conventional OADR, we can see that it is not"?

Here, we have what is known as Segall's Law. Lee Segall bought a radio station in Dallas, Texas, in the early days of that medium and created the world's first quiz show. He is reputed to have said, "A man with a watch knows what time it is. A man with two watches is never sure" (Strange Wondrous 2008). In discussions of population aging, it is difficult to entertain two conceptually similar measures, such as the OADR and the POADR, that show such different speeds of aging. Inevitably, people will have to choose.

The conventional measures and the prospective ones differ in only one way; they use different old-age thresholds. Thus, the choice between the conventional and the prospective measures provided in *World Population Ageing 2017* boils down to which old-age threshold is preferable: one that is constant over time, space, and all population subgroups, or one that takes the remaining life expectancy of people into account. In other words, it is the choice of which glasses to use. In this chapter, we examine the choice between the two. First, we will discuss the philosophical and conceptual differences. Next, we will very briefly review some historical and forecasted values of life expectancy. Finally, we will assess the difficulty of switching from the old glasses to the new ones.

Philosophical and Conceptual Differences

At its most fundamental level, the choice of whether to use prospective measures or conventional ones depends on how we think about people. Conventional measures ignore differences in how people function at age 65, or some other fixed chronological age, and use that fixed age to mark the onset of old age regardless of any other factor. Prospective measures, on the other hand, use a different concept of age, one related to remaining life expectancy, a factor correlated with functional ability, and one that varies over time, space, and population subgroups. The choice of which of the old-age dependency ratios on the United Nations' website to use depends on which view of people is adopted.

Differences in Remaining Life Expectancy

Is it plausible to believe that the stage of old age begins at age 65 all over the world and for the entire period from 1950–1955 to 2095–2100? To assess the reasonableness of this assumption, we can look at remaining life expectancies from the United Nations' estimates and forecasts on the assumption that old age universally begins at age 65. We show the result for a variety of countries in Table 13.1. We must conclude that 65-year-old Chinese in 1950–1955 entered old age with a remaining life expectancy of 8.72 years, while 65-year-old Japanese in 2095–2100 will enter old age when they have a remaining life expectancy of 29.80 years. It seems implausible to us that people with a remaining

Table 13.1   Remaining life expectancy (both sexes) at age 65

	1950–1955	2095–2100
Canada	14.39	28.17
Chile	12.87	27.12
China	8.72	24.09
Costa Rica	12.30	27.17
Egypt	12.69	21.20
France	13.52	28.94
India	9.80	20.08
Japan	12.51	29.80
South Africa	11.36	19.78

Data source: United Nations (2017e).

life expectancy of 8.72 years and 29.80 years should be assumed to be equally old or to have equal functional ability. In contrast, the prospective measures classify people as being equally old based on their remaining life expectancy. Throughout this book, we have presented our arguments and those of others that characteristics matter in assessing aging. It is certainly convenient, from an administrative perspective, to use age 65 as an old-age threshold, but we do not know of anyone or any statistical agency that makes the argument that it is plausible that 65-year-olds are equally elderly everywhere in the world.

Differences in the Difficulty of Use

We have argued in this book that prospective measures of population aging enable us to see past and possible future patterns of population aging more clearly, but, before we recommend their use, we have to discuss whether there are any difficulties of doing so. Up to now, there have been three main issues related to the use of our measures. Most importantly, the difficulties associated with deviating from what the United Nations published. Now that *World Population Ageing 2017* (United Nations 2017a, 2017e) incorporates our POADRs, there is no longer any cost of deviating from what the United Nations publishes. The second difficulty had arisen because of ease of access. Now, however, our POADRs are published in *World Population Ageing 2017* along with all the other measures of aging they are familiar with using. Prospective measures of population aging can also be found on our website, www.reaging.org. So, the problem of where to find prospective measures of aging has also vanished.

One disadvantage of using prospective measures of aging remains. The conventional measures categorize people as being old starting at age 65. The prospective measures categorize people as being old when they get to the age where remaining life expectancy is 15 years. It is harder for many people to understand the meaning of "the age where remaining life expectancy is 15 years" than to understand "age 65." The old glasses have been in use so long that people are thoroughly familiar with them. It will undoubtedly take some time for them to become equally comfortable with the new ones, the ones that the United Nations has now made much more easily accessible.

Which Glasses to Wear

Different pairs of glasses can be worn for different purposes. Some are for reading and some are for driving. What the United Nations has done is to say that our glasses are appropriate to wear for some purposes. There is no cost to trying them on. We believe that they will make your perception of population aging much clearer. If you do not like them, you can always put the old ones back on.

Conclusion

OUR LAST STOP is a renovated palace around 11 miles (17 kilometers) south of Vienna, Austria. The palace, known as Schloss Laxenburg, is where most of the research for this book was done. Our office is on the ground floor looking out on a beautiful park. The palace was built in the 1750s during the reign of Empress Maria Theresa. She had 16 children, 10 of whom survived to adulthood. They and their descendants became an important component of European aristocracy in their day. Perhaps the two most famous of them were the ill-fated Marie Antoinette and Joseph II, who became Holy Roman Emperor from 1765 to 1780. They played right out there in the park. Emperor Franz Joseph often stayed here with his wife, Elisabeth. The room overlooking the park where they had breakfast has been reconstructed and is just upstairs. The palace now houses the International Institute for Applied Systems Analysis where researchers from all over the world come together to study global problems. Please join us here for a cup of coffee and a delicious Austrian pastry. We have covered quite a bit of territory in this book and, before we part, it would be pleasant to sit for a while and discuss what we have seen and what still remains to be explored.

This book is like a new pair of glasses with a better prescription. The new vision allows us to see more clearly what is around us. The additional clarity of our vision results from our enlargement of the concept of age from a unidimensional one to a multidimensional one. If we were to ask a 70-year-old woman how old she is, she would tell us she was 70 years old. If we were to ask her how "elderly" she was, she might tell us that she is not elderly at all, that she still regularly attends yoga classes, that she delivers meals to older people who cannot shop for themselves, and that she runs the website for her church. She might tell us that she and her husband have a comfortable life; that last summer they spent 2 weeks in the Canadian Rockies with their children and grandchildren; and this coming December she and her husband were planning on spending some time in Vienna, going to the opera and enjoying the wonderful outdoor markets that pop up at that time of year. How old the woman is and how elderly she is are two very different things. When we had our old pair of glasses on, the ones that were originally constructed around a century ago, we could not distinguish between how old she was and how elderly she was. Now with our new glasses, we can.

People have many characteristics that are germane to the study of population aging and these characteristics are different in different places, change from one population subgroup to another, and vary over time. When we tell people that this is the core idea of our book, they often look at us quizzically and respond with a question which is some version of "Doesn't everyone know this?" and the follow-up question sometimes is, "Why are you writing a book about something that everyone knows?" The answer is that everyone does know this, but that this knowledge has not been reflected in published statistics and therefore is usually ignored in public and policy discussions.

This mismatch between what everyone knows and how measures of population aging have been computed has been growing and, with our old glasses, our vision of the demographic environment has become significantly occluded. The old glasses were comfortable, and up to now no one had offered an alternative pair. But this has now changed. In our research and in this book, we have offered an alternative pair of glasses and the United Nations Population Division, having perceived the mismatch, has tried them on. Our *prospective old-age dependency ratio (POADR)* now is available for all United Nations countries on their website (United Nations 2017f).

Our POADR is only one of the interesting features of the demographic environment that we saw when wearing the new pair of glasses. In this book, we presented many more. Although, we have been wearing the new glasses for a while now, we ourselves keep being pleasantly surprised by all the new things that we can see. Our first surprise came in Sanderson and Scherbov (2005), where we saw that over time the *prospective median age* of a population can decrease, even as the conventional one increases. We showed some examples of this in Chapter 4. Later, when we defined measures of population aging using our *prospective old-age threshold*, we also saw observations like those for Northern Europe, where the OADR went up and the POADR went down. We also showed examples of this in Chapter 4.

Our initial research was focused around the implications of people having *prospective ages*, prospective old-age thresholds, and *constant characteristic ages*. Later, we were surprised when we learned that our newly widened vision was still too narrow, and we developed the concept of α-*ages*. Prospective age is an age based on remaining life expectancy, but the same reasoning that we used to produce prospective ages could be used to produce ages based on many characteristics (Sanderson and Scherbov 2013). We discussed α-ages in Chapter 5, using as pertinent characteristics, the 5-year survival rate and the *life course ratio*. The life course ratio at each age is the fraction of adult lifetimes that are spent at that age and above. The life course ratio is a natural measure for demographers to study because it is available in life tables and provides an interesting way of looking at aging.

Much attention has been given to the remaining life expectancy of older people, particularly to the adjustment of pension payouts to changes in it. But aging needs to be studied both in terms of remaining life expectancy and the proportion of people who survive to the given life expectancies. We initially introduced the life course ratio in order to have a measure of aging that incorporated both of those aspects. Later, we were surprised to discover that our intergenerationally equitable pension age was a constant characteristic age and that the characteristic was not remaining life expectancy but the life course ratio (Sanderson and Scherbov 2015a).

There were elements in almost every chapter of this book that surprised us. The most surprising, though, was our finding, discussed in

Chapter 10, that faster increases in life expectancy led to slower population aging (Sanderson and Scherbov 2015b). Hundreds of books, articles, and websites say the opposite. In a one-dimensional world, where
old age is assumed to begin at age 65, they are correct, but, when we
take the changing characteristics of people into account, things look
different. If scientists are successful in slowing the aging process, tomorrow's 65-year-olds will not be like today's 65-year-olds; they will
be functionally younger. With our new glasses, we can see this. A detailed mathematical explanation of why faster increases in life expectancy lead to slower population aging can be found in Ediev, Sanderson,
and Scherbov (2019).

As we hiked around the demographic environment, looking at all
the new and interesting features of population aging that were now visible to us, we were struck by how sparsely populated the area was. The
measurement of population aging has not been a topic of study, despite
its importance. It is typically only mentioned in passing in textbooks
and in courses in demography and its history is largely ignored. Time
after time seminal contributions have been forgotten and had to be reinvented and there may well be other contributions that remain forgotten. This is particularly striking because of the difficulty of de-
fending the current practice of focusing on measures that are based
only on people's chronological ages.

We do not know why the measurement of population aging has not
become a topic of study, but we conjecture that there may be three reasons. First, measures of population aging based solely on characteristics that do not change over time already exist. These measures have
been produced by many statistical agencies, so unless one disagrees
with those measures, there is no incentive to devise or even think
about new ones. Second, those measures have not been interesting from
a methodological standpoint. They are simple ratios or medians. Finally, the United Nations and other statistical agencies have produced
what are the de facto standard numbers. It is much easier for people to
discuss a phenomenon like population aging, when they are all using
the same numbers.

But now things are different. The United Nations' website on aging
now has two old-age dependency ratios. No longer is the conventional
old-age dependency ratio the sole standard. Beyond that, in this book,

we have shown that there are a wide variety of interesting aspects of aging that can be seen when the old, one-dimensional glasses are discarded and the new ones are worn.

As much new territory as we have explored together, there still remains much more yet to explore. We have only noted tangentially the inequality across population subgroups in patterns of aging. Much has been written about this by others (Marmot 2005; Marmot et al. 2008; Brunner et al. 2009; Gallo et al. 2012; Nabi et al. 2008; Mackenbach 2012; Rautio, Heikkinen, and Ebrahim 2005; OECD 2017) and we have written a few related papers (Ghislandi, Sanderson, and Scherbov 2019; Sanderson and Scherbov 2014, 2016; Sanderson et al. 2016) on the topic. It is an important area to explore further, but it would have taken us too far afield here.

We have not explored population aging through the use of microsimulation models. This has been done in the Future Elderly Model (FEM) (Roybal Center for Health Policy Simulation, n.d.), a complex demographic-economic microsimulation model. The model was developed originally for the United States and has now been adapted to a few more countries. The model is very wide-ranging, allowing researchers to investigate a variety of policy questions regarding aging in the country being modeled, including those dealing with inequality and financial costs. On fundamental issues, our view is roughly consistent with what the FEM sees. The FEM website states,

> Researchers used the FEM to predict life expectancy, and then used regression analyses to compare the predictive power of the two variables in explaining health care expenditures. Age has little additional predictive power on health care expenditures after controlling for life expectancy. (Roybal Center for Health Policy Simulation, n.d.)

Nevertheless, a full discussion and evaluation of complex microsimulation models full of country-specific institutional details was also beyond what we could explore here.

We could also not explore the financial sustainability of countries' fiscal arrangements. Exciting new work in this area is being done in the context of the National Transfer Accounts (NTA) project (NTA, n.d.a). Exploring the linkages between NTA results and ours is an intriguing direction for future research.

When public policies are designed to take the changing characteristics of people into account, sustainability will be enhanced, but we have not done the calculations for individual countries. Even during the writing of this book, pension age policies in a number of countries have changed, so those sorts of calculations are likely to quickly become out of date. Our interest here was not to give policy advice to specific countries but to provide a new demographic framework for the formulation of policies related to population aging.

Nevertheless, our view does have an important implication for fiscal sustainability. If public policies regarding the elderly are written in terms of fixed chronological ages, with increasing life expectancies an ever-greater proportion of the population will either be eligible or almost eligible for benefits or have a family member who is. For example, if pension benefits are defined using a fixed chronological age, a growing proportion of the population will have a financial interest in maintaining or expanding those benefits. As a result, the political pressure to maintain unsustainable pension policies is likely to increase (Sanderson and Scherbov 2007). Seeing population aging more clearly can help prevent this and play a role in keeping countries fiscally sound.

It is time to say goodbye. We have traveled far together and seen many interesting things. Your new glasses are yours to keep. You have a choice. You can wear them or put the old ones back on. We hope that you will keep the new ones on and join us in continuing to explore the beautiful and interesting multidimensional world of population aging.

GLOSSARY

Age differences These are the differences between α-*ages* and chronological ages. *Age differences* measure differences in variables related to aging between a population of interest and a *standard population* and express those differences in years of age regardless of how the underlying variables are measured.

Age difference trajectories These trajectories are *age differences* arrayed by chronological age.

α-*ages* These are ages based on characteristics of people. α-*ages* are always comparative.

α-*age of someone of chronological age x* This is the age in the *standard population* where people have the same level of some characteristic as people of chronological age x in the population of interest.

α-*gender gaps in survival* These are differences between *age difference trajectories* for men and for women. The age difference trajectories use the country with the highest survival rates as the standard country. The resulting age difference trajectories quantify how far each gender is behind best-practice. α-*gender gaps in survival* quantify how far women are behind their best practice survival rates compared to how far men are behind theirs.

Characteristics approach to the study of population aging This is the approach to the study of population aging developed by Sanderson and Scherbov and used in this book.

Characteristic schedule This is the relationship between the level of a specific characteristic and chronological age.

Constant characteristic age This is the age in a population where people have some fixed level of a characteristic (for example, average hand-grip strength).

Conventional old-age threshold The *conventional old-age threshold* is usually set at age 60 or 65 and does not change over time, over space, or across population subgroups. People at or above the conventional old-age threshold are categorized as being old.

Conventional proportion of adult lifetimes spent in old age (PALO) This is the proportion of person-years lived from age 20 onward that are also lived at or beyond the *conventional old-age threshold*.

Economic support ratio (ESR) This is based on data created in the National Transfer Accounts (NTA) project and merges standard economic accounts with life cycle generational accounting. It is computed as the ratio of the number of standardized producers to the number of standardized consumers.

Intergenerationally equitable normal pension age This is the pension age where each generation is treated equitably, even as survival conditions change. Using the *intergenerationally equitable pension age,* no cohort subsidizes another. The intergenerationally equitable pension age is a *constant characteristic age* where the characteristic is the *life course ratio.*

Life course ratio (at age x) This is the fraction of all *person-years lived* from age 20 onward that are also lived from age x onward.

Life expectancy schedules These are tables or graphs that show the relationship between chronological age and *remaining life expectancy.*

Median age (MA) The *median age* is a conventional measure of population aging. It is the age that divides a population into two numerically equal groups, with half of the people being younger than this age and half older.

Old-age dependency ratio (OADR) The *old-age dependency ratio* is a conventional measure of population aging. In this book, it is usually defined as the ratio of people 65 years old or older to the ratio of those between 20 and 64 years old. When statistical agencies present this ratio, it is often multiplied by 100.

Person-years lived from age x onward This is the total number of years people who have survived to age x live from that age onward. It is computed using the age-specific mortality rates of a given period or cohort. The average number of person-years lived from age x onward by people who have survived to age x is *remaining life expectancy at age x*.

Population A population is a group of people. While individuals who are still alive grow older each year, populations can grow either older or younger. Whether a population is growing older or younger is assessed using measures of population aging. It is possible for a population to grow older when using conventional measures of aging and younger when using prospective measures. This illustrates the multidimensional nature of population aging.

Population projections Estimates of future population size and composition based on assumptions about future trends in fertility, mortality, and migration.

Proportion of the population categorized as being old (PO) This is a conventional measure of population aging. It is the share of the population above the *conventional old-age threshold*. Usually this age is either 60 or 65.

Proportion of the 65+ population who are categorized as old (P65O) This is the proportion of the population who are 65 or more years old who are also at or above the *prospective old-age threshold*.

Prospective The adjective *prospective* is used to denote any measure of population aging that is based on remaining life expectancy. Specific examples of its use follow.

Prospective ages These are a special case of α-*ages* where the characteristic is remaining life expectancy.

Prospective age of someone of chronological age x This is the age in the *standard population* where people have the same remaining life expectancy as people of chronological age x in the population of interest.

Prospective constant characteristic age This is a *constant characteristic age* where the characteristic is remaining life expectancy.

Prospective median age (PMA) This is the age in a *standard population* where people have the same remaining life expectancy as people in the population being studied have at their median age.

Prospective old-age dependency ratio (POADR) The *prospective old-age dependency ratio* is defined as the ratio of people at or above the *prospective old-age-threshold* to those from age 20 to the prospective old-age threshold.

Prospective old-age threshold (POAT) This is a flexible threshold age defining the group of people who are categorized as old. It assumes that people are not categorized as old based only on a fixed chronological age. Instead, this old-age threshold depends on characteristics of people. In this book, the *prospective old-age threshold* is the age at which remaining life expectancy first falls below 15 years.

Prospective proportion of adult lifetimes spent in old age (PPALO) This is the proportion of person-years lived from age 20 onward that are also lived at or beyond the *prospective old-age threshold*.

Prospective proportion who are considered old (PPO) This is the proportion of the population at or above the *prospective old-age threshold*.

Remaining life expectancy at age 65 (same as life expectancy at age 65) This is the average number of years a 65-year-old person has left to live for the rest of his or her life if subjected to the age-specific mortality rates of a given period or cohort.

Remaining life expectancy at age x (same as life expectancy at age x) This is the average number of years a x-year-old person has left to live for the rest of his or her life if subjected to the age-specific mortality rates of a given period or cohort. This definition is appropriate for any age x.

Standard population (standard country/standard schedule) *Characteristic schedules* from the *standard population* are used for comparison in the computation of *prospective ages, prospective median ages, α-ages, age differences, age difference trajectories,* and *α-gender gap trajectories.*

Total dependency ratio (TDR) The *total dependency ratio* is the ratio of those classified as dependents to those classified as potential supporters.

REFERENCES

Agenta. n.d. "AGENTA project." Accessed November 13, 2017. http://www
.agenta-project.eu/en/index.htm.

Al Snih, Soham, Kyriakos S. Markides, Kenneth J. Ottenbacher, and Mukaila A.
Raji. 2004. "Hand Grip Strength and Incident ADL Disability in Elderly Mex-
ican Americans over a Seven-Year Period." *Aging Clinical and Experimental
Research* 16, no. 6: 481–486. https://doi.org/10.1007/BF03327406.

Anstey, Kaarin J., Mary A. Luszcz, Lynne C. Giles, and Gary R. Andrews. 2001.
"Demographic, Health, Cognitive, and Sensory Variables as Predictors of Mortality in Very Old Adults." *Psychology and Aging* 16, no. 1: 3–11. https://doi
.org/10.1037/0882-7974.16.1.3.

Balabkins, Nicholas W. 1978. "Der Zukunftsstaat: Carl Ballod's Vision of a
Leisure-Oriented Socialism." *History of Political Economy* 10, no. 2: 213–232.
https://doi.org/10.1215/00182702-10-2-213.

Ballod, Carl. 1913. *Grundriss Der Statistik: Enthaltend Bevoelkerungs-,
Wirtschafts-, Finanz- Und Handels-Statistik.* Berlin: J. Guttentag.

Barslund, Mikkel C., and Marten von Werder. 2017. "Measuring Dependency Ratios
Using National Transfer Accounts." *Vienna Yearbook of Population Research*
2016, no. 14: 155–186. https://doi.org/10.1553/populationyearbook2016s155.

Bohannon, Richard W. 2001. "Dynamometer Measurements of Hand-Grip
Strength Predict Multiple Outcomes." *Perceptual and Motor Skills* 93, no. 2:
323–328. https://doi.org/10.2466/pms.2001.93.2.323.

Bordone, Valeria, Sergei Scherbov, and Nadia Steiber. 2015. "Smarter Every Day:
The Deceleration of Population Ageing in Terms of Cognition." *Intelligence*
52 (September): 90–96. https://doi.org/10.1016/j.intell.2015.07.005.

Börsch-Supan, Axel, Martina Brandt, Christian Hunkler, Thorsten Kneip, Julie
Korbmacher, Frederic Malter, Barbara Schaan, Stephanie Stuck, and Sabrina
Zuber. 2013. "Data Resource Profile: The Survey of Health, Ageing and Re-
tirement in Europe (SHARE)." *International Journal of Epidemiology* 42, no. 4
(August): 992–1001. https://doi.org/10.1093/ije/dyt088.

Bourdelais, Patrick. 1998. "The Ageing of the Population: Relevant Question or
Obsolete Matter." In *Old Age from Antiquity to Post-modernity,* edited by
Paul Johnson and Pat Thane, 110–131. London: Routledge.

Bronikowski, Anne M., Jeanne Altmann, Diane K. Brockman, Marina Cords, Linda M. Fedigan, Anne Pusey, Tara Stoinski, William F. Morris, Karen B. Strier, and Susan C. Alberts. 2011. "Aging in the Natural World: Comparative Data Reveal Similar Mortality Patterns across Primates." *Science* 331, no. 6022: 1325–1328. https://doi.org/10.1126/science.1201571.

Brueck, Hilary. 2018. "A 69-Year-Old Dutch Man Just Tried to Legally Subtract 20 Years from His Age—but the Court Said No Way." *Business Insider Deutschland*, December 3, 2018. https://www.businessinsider.de/dutchman -emile-ratelband-wants-to-legally-change-his-age-2018-11?r=US&IR=T.

Brunner, Eric, Martin Shipley, Victoria Spencer, Mika Kivimaki, Tarani Chandola, David Gimeno, Archana Singh-Manoux, Jack Guralnik, and Michael Marmot. 2009. "Social Inequality in Walking Speed in Early Old Age in the Whitehall II Study." *Journals of Gerontology Series A* 64A, no. 10 (October): 1082–1089. https://doi.org/10.1093/gerona/glp078.

Bussolo, Maurizio, Johannes Koettl, and Emily Sinnott. 2015. "Golden Aging: Prospects for Healthy, Active, and Prosperous Aging in Europe and Central Asia." In *Europe and Central Asia Studies*. Washington, DC: World Bank. https://openknowledge.worldbank.org/bitstream/handle/10986/22018/97814 64803536.pdf.

Cigna. 2015a. "Data Appendix: Understanding the over 50s Market in 2015 Britain." Accessed October 19, 2017. https://www.cignainsure.co.uk/sites/cigna _insure/files/public/Cigna%20Insurance%20Services%20Corporate%20 Deck%20September%202015%20Data%20Appendix.pdf.

———. 2015b. "It's Official: 'Life Now Begins at 60' According to New Research Middle Age Stretches as Far as 68 for Young at Heart Baby Boomers." November 6, 2015. Accessed October 19, 2017. https://www.cignainsurance.co.uk/media-centre /press-announcements/life-now-begins-at-60-according-to-new-Cigna-research.

———. 2015c. "Understanding the over 50s Market in 2015 Britain." Accessed October 19, 2017. https://www.cignainsure.co.uk/life-begins-at-60.

Cole, William E., and S. E. T. Lund. 1941. "The Tennessee River Valley, Its People, Resources, and Institutions." *Journal of Educational Sociology* 15, no. 3: 130–136. https://doi.org/10.2307/2261755.

Cooper, Rachel, Bjorn Heine Strand, Rebecca Hardy, Kushang V. Patel, and Diana Kuh. 2014. "Physical Capability in Mid-life and Survival over 13 Years of Follow-Up: British Birth Cohort Study." *British Medical Journal* 348 (April): g2219. https://doi.org/10.1136/bmj.g2219.

Cutler, David M., James M. Poterba, Lawrence M. Sheiner, Louise H. Summers, and George A. Akerlof. 1990. "An Aging Society: Opportunity or Challenge?" *Brookings Papers on Economic Activity* 1990, no. 1: 1–73. https://doi.org/10 .2307/2534525.

Daw, R. H. 1961. "The Comparison of Male and Female Mortality Rates." *Journal of the Royal Statistical Society. Series A (General)* 124, no. 1: 20–43. https://doi .org/10.2307/2343151.

Domonoske, Camila. 2018. "Dutch Man Loses Bid to Change His Age, Plans to Appeal." *NPR*, December 4, 2018. https://www.npr.org/2018/12/04/673246844 /dutch-man-loses-bid-to-change-his-age-plans-to-appeal?t=1548346774106.

Ediev, Dalkhat M., Warren C. Sanderson, and Sergei Scherbov. 2019. "The Formal Demography of Prospective Age: The Relationship between the Old-Age Dependency Ratio and the Prospective Old-Age Dependency Ratio." *Theoretical Population Biology* 125 (February): 1–10. https://www.sciencedirect.com /science/article/pii/S004058091730120X.

EHLEIS (European Health and Life Expectancy Information System). n.d.a. "European Health and Life Expectancy Information System." Accessed November 9, 2017. http://www.eurohex.eu/.

———. n.d.b. "SHARE Question on Instrumental Activities of Daily Living." Montpellier, France: French National Institute of Health and Medical Research. Accessed October 30, 2017. http://www.eurohex.eu/ehleis/metadata /Metadata_SHARE_IADL.pdf.

———. n.d.c. "SHARE Question on Physical Functional Limitation." Montpellier, France: French National Institute of Health and Medical Research. Accessed October 30, 2017. http://www.eurohex.eu/ehleis/metadata/Metadata_SHARE _PFL.pdf.

Eurostat. 2017. "A Look at the Lives of the Elderly in the EU Today." Luxembourg: European Commission. http://ec.europa.eu/eurostat/cache/infographs/elderly /index.html.

Federal State Statistics Service, Russian Federation. n.d. "Интерактивная Витрина." Accessed August 11, 2017. http://cbsd.gks.ru.

Fuchs, Victor R. 1984. "'Though Much Is Taken': Reflections on Aging, Health, and Medical Care." *Milbank Memorial Fund Quarterly-Health and Society* 62, no. 2: 143–166.

Fukumori, Norio, Yosuke Yamamoto, Misa Takegami, Shin Yamazaki, Yoshihiro Onishi, Miho Sekiguchi, Koji Otani, Shin-ichi Konno, Shin-ichi Kikuchi, and Shunichi Fukuhara. 2015. "Association between Hand-Grip Strength and Depressive Symptoms: Locomotive Syndrome and Health Outcomes in Aizu Cohort Study (LOHAS)." *Age and Ageing* 44, no. 4: 592–598. https://doi.org /10.1093/ageing/afv013.

Gallo, Valentina, Johan P. Mackenbach, Majid Ezzati, Gwenn Menvielle, Anton E. Kunst, Sabine Rohrmann, Rudolf Kaaks, et al. 2012. "Social Inequalities and Mortality in Europe—Results from a Large Multi-National Cohort." *PLoS ONE* 7, no. 7 (July 25): e39013. https://doi.org/10.1371/journal .pone.0039013.

Ghislandi, Simone, Warren C. Sanderson, and Sergei Scherbov. 2019. "A Simple Measure of Human Development: The Human Life Indicator." *Population and Development Review* 45, no. 1 (March): 219–233. https://doi.org/10.1111 /padr.12205.

Groom, Nelson. 2015. "Watch Out Usain Bolt! Meet the 105-Year-Old Sprinter Who Just Set a 100-Metre World Record . . . in 42.22 Seconds." *Daily Mail*, September 25, 2015. http://www.dailymail.co.uk/news/article-3248469/World -s-oldest-competitive-sprinter-sets-new-sprinting-record.html.

Grund, Ashley, and Aimee Lewis. 2017. "World Masters Games: Man Kaur Wins 100m Gold—Aged 101." CNN, April 26, 2017. http://edition.cnn.com/2017/04 /25/sport/101-year-old-man-kaur-wins-100m-world-masters-games/.

Günther, Ernst. 1931. "Der Geburtenrückgang als Ursache der Arbeitslosigkeit? Untersuchung einiger Zusammenhänge zwischen Wirtschaft und Bevölkerungsbewegung." *Jahrbücher für Nationalökonomie und Statistik*: 921–973.

Hanten, William P., Wen-Yin Chen, Alicia Ann Austin, Rebecca E. Brooks, Harlan Clay Carter, Carol Ann Law, Melanie Kay Morgan, Donna Jean Sanders, Christe Ann Swan, and Amy Lorraine Vanderslice. 1999. "Maximum Grip Strength in Normal Subjects from 20 to 64 Years of Age." *Journal of Hand Therapy* 12, no. 3: 193–200. https://doi.org/10.1016/S0894-1130(99)80046-5.

He, Wan, Daniel Goodkind, Paul Kowal, and United States Census Bureau. 2016. "An Aging World: 2015." International Population Reports P95 / 16-1. Washington, DC: US Government Publishing Office. http://www.census.gov/content/dam/Census/library/publications/2016/demo/p95-16-1.pdf.

Himmer, Alastair. 2015. "Twinkle-Toed Japan Sprinter Still Breaking Records at 105." L'Agence France-Presse (AFP), October 29, 2015. https://correspondent.afp.com/twinkle-toed-japan-sprinter-still-breaking-records-105.

HRS (Health and Retirement Study). n.d. "Health and Retirement Study." Accessed November 9, 2017. https://hrs.isr.umich.edu/about/international-sister-studies.

Hutt, Rosamond. 2016. "In Which Countries Do Women Outlive Men by More than a Decade?" World Economic Forum. https://www.weforum.org/agenda/2016/05/countries-where-women-outlive-men-by-decade/.

Japan Times Online. 2015. "Senior Sprinter Dubbed 'Golden Bolt' Sets World Record." September 23, 2015. http://www.japantimes.co.jp/sports/2015/09/23/more-sports/track-field/senior-sprinter-dubbed-golden-bolt-sets-world-record/.

Kemper, Steve. 2013. "Humans Would Be Better Off If They Monkeyed Around Like the Muriquis." *Smithsonian Magazine*, September 2013. https://www.smithsonianmag.com/science-nature/humans-would-be-better-off-if-they-monkeyed-around-like-the-muriquis-833014/.

Koopman, Jacob J. E., David van Bodegom, Diana van Heemst, and Rudi G. J. Westendorp. 2015. "Handgrip Strength, Ageing and Mortality in Rural Africa." *Age and Ageing* 44, no. 3: 465–470. https://doi.org/10.1093/ageing/afu165.

Lee, Ronald, and Joshua R. Goldstein. 2003. "Rescaling the Life Cycle: Longevity and Proportionality." In "Life Span: Evolutionary, Ecological, and Demographic Perspectives," edited by J. R. Carey and S. Tuljapurkar, supplement, *Population and Development Review* 29: 183–207. http://www.jstor.org/stable/3401351.

Ling, Carolina H. Y., Diana Taekema, Anton J. M. de Craen, Jacobijn Gussekloo, Rudi G. J. Westendorp, and Andrea B. Maier. 2010. "Handgrip Strength and Mortality in the Oldest Old Population: The Leiden 85-Plus Study." *Canadian Medical Association Journal* 182, no. 5: 429–435. https://doi.org/10.1503/cmaj.091278.

Lowsky, David J., S. Jay Olshansky, Jay Bhattacharya, and Dana P. Goldman. 2014. "Heterogeneity in Healthy Aging." *Journals of Gerontology Series A:*

Biological Sciences and Medical Sciences 69, no. 6 (June 1): 640–649. https://doi .org/10.1093/gerona/glt162.

Lutz, Wolfgang, Warren C. Sanderson, and Sergei Scherbov. 2008. "The Coming Acceleration of Global Population Ageing." *Nature* 451, no. 7179: 716–719. https://doi.org/10.1038/nature06516.

Luy, Marc. 2003. "Causes of Male Excess Mortality: Insights from Cloistered Populations." *Population and Development Review* 29, no. 4: 647–676. https://doi .org/10.1111/j.1728-4457.2003.00647.x.

Mackenbach, Johan P. 2012. "The Persistence of Health Inequalities in Modern Welfare States: The Explanation of a Paradox." *Social Science and Medicine* 75, no. 4: 761–769. https://doi.org/10.1016/j.socscimed.2012.02.031.

Marmot, Michael. 2005. "Social Determinants of Health Inequalities." *Lancet* 365, no. 9464: 1099–1104. https://doi.org/10.1016/S0140-6736(05)71146-6.

Marmot, Michael G., Martin J. Shipley, Harry Hemingway, Jenny Head, and Eric J. Brunner. 2008. "Biological and Behavioural Explanations of Social Inequalities in Coronary Heart Disease: The Whitehall II Study." *Diabetologia* 51, no. 11: 1980. https://doi.org/10.1007/s00125-008-1144-3.

Mason, Andrew, Ronald Lee, Michael Abrigo, Sang-Hyop Lee. 2017. "Support Ratios and Demographic Dividends: Estimates for the World." Technical Paper No. 2017/1. United Nations Department of Economic and Social Affairs, New York.

Memoires de L'Academie Imperiale des Sciences de St. Pétersbourg. 1897. Vol. 8, ser. 1, no. 5. Saint Petersburg: L'Academie.

Milligan, Kevin S., and David A. Wise. 2011. "Social Security and Retirement around the World: Historical Trends in Mortality and Health, Employment, and Disability Insurance Participation and Reforms—Introduction and Summary." Working Paper 16719, National Bureau of Economic Research (January). https://doi.org/10.3386/w16719.

MPIDR (Max Planck Institute for Demographic Research). n.d. "Max Planck Research Group: Gender Gaps in Health and Survival." Accessed January 8, 2019. https://www.demogr.mpg.de/en/laboratories/gender_gaps_in_health _and_survival_3860/projects/default.htm.

Nabi, Hermann, Mika Kivimaki, Michael G. Marmot, Jane Ferrie, Marie Zins, Pierre Ducimetiere, Silla M. Consoli, and Archana Singh-Manoux. 2008. "Does Personality Explain Social Inequalities in Mortality? The French GAZEL Cohort Study." *International Journal of Epidemiology* 37, no. 3: 591–602. https://doi.org/10.1093/ije/dyn021.

Neugarten, Bernice L. *The Meanings of Age: Selected Papers.* Chicago: University of Chicago Press, 1996.

Notestein, Frank W., Irene B. Taeuber, Dudley Kirk, Ansley J. Coale, and Louise K. Kiser. 1944. *The Future Population of Europe and the Soviet Union: Population Projections 1940–1970.* Vol. 2. Geneva: League of Nations.

NTA (National Transfer Accounts). n.d.a. "National Transfer Accounts Project." Accessed October 9, 2017. http://www.ntaccounts.org/web/nta/show/.

———. n.d.b. "Gender, Time Use." Accessed November 13, 2017. http://www .ntaccounts.org/web/nta/show/Gender,%20Time%20use.

―――. n.d.c. "National Transfer Accounts Project: NTA Data." Accessed November 8, 2017. http://www.ntaccounts.org/web/nta/show/NTA%20Data.

―――. n.d.d. "National Transfer Accounts: Understanding the Generational Economy." Accessed November 8, 2017. http://www.ntaccounts.org/web/nta/show.

OECD (Organisation for Economic Co-operation and Development). 2013. *Pensions at a Glance 2013: Retirement-Income Systems in OECD and G20 Countries*. Paris: OECD Publishing. http://www.oecd.org/pensions/pensionsataglance.htm.

―――. 2015. *Pensions at a Glance 2015: OECD and G20 Indicators*. Paris: OECD Publishing. http://dx.doi.org/10.1787/pension_glance-2015-en.

―――. 2016. "Elderly Population." Paris: Organisation for Economic Co-operation and Development. https://data.oecd.org/pop/elderly-population.htm.

―――. 2017. "Preventing Ageing Unequally." Paris: OECD Publishing. http://dx.doi.org/10.1787/9789264279087-en.

Race Against Time Foundation. 2017. "Palo Alto Longevity Prize." August 14, 2017. http://paloaltoprize.com/.

Raftery, Adrian E., Nan Li, Hana Ševčíková, Patrick Gerland, and Gerhard K. Heilig. 2012. "Bayesian Probabilistic Population Projections for All Countries." *Proceedings of the National Academy of Sciences* 109, no. 35: 13915–13921. https://doi.org/10.1073/pnas.1211452109.

RANEPA (Russian Presidential Academy of National Economy and Public Administration), Rosstat (Russian Federal State Statistics Service), and IIASA (International Institute for Applied Systems Analysis). 2016. "Russian Demographic Data Sheet 2016." Moscow, Russia, and Laxenburg, Austria: RANEPA, Rosstat, IIASA. http://www.iiasa.ac.at/web/home/research/researchPrograms/WorldPopulation/PublicationsMediaCoverage/ModelsData/Russian_DataSheet_web.pdf.

Rapoza, Kenneth. 2017. "China's Aging Population Becoming More of a Problem." *Forbes*, February 21, 2017. https://www.forbes.com/sites/kenrapoza/2017/02/21/chinas-aging-population-becoming-more-of-a-problem/#cb68f4a140f3.

Rautio, Nina, Eino Heikkinen, and Shah Ebrahim. 2005. "Socio-economic Position and Its Relationship to Physical Capacity among Elderly People Living in Jyväskylä, Finland: Five- and Ten-Year Follow-Up Studies." *Social Science and Medicine (1982)* 60, no. 11: 2405–2416. https://doi.org/10.1016/j.socscimed.2004.11.029.

REVES (Réseau Espérance de Vie en Santé). n.d. "Network on Health Expectancy and the Disability Process." Accessed November 9, 2017. https://reves.site.ined.fr/en/home.

Roberts, Helen C., Hayley J. Denison, Helen J. Martin, Harnish P. Patel, Holly Syddall, Cyrus Cooper, and Avan Aihie Sayer. 2011. "A Review of the Measurement of Grip Strength in Clinical and Epidemiological Studies: Towards a Standardised Approach." *Age and Ageing* 40, no. 4: 423–429. https://doi.org/10.1093/ageing/afr051.

Roybal Center for Health Policy Simulation. n.d. "The Future Elderly Model." Accessed January 2, 2019. https://roybalhealthpolicy.usc.edu/fem/#value delayedaging.

Ryder, Norman B. 1975. "Notes on Stationary Populations." *Population Index* 41, no. 1: 3–28. https://doi.org/10.2307/2734140.

Sanderson, Warren C., and Sergei Scherbov. 2005. "Average Remaining Lifetimes Can Increase as Human Populations Age." *Nature* 435, no. 7043: 811–813. https://doi.org/10.1038/nature03593.

———. 2007a. "A Near Electoral Majority of Pensioners: Prospects and Policies." *Population and Development Review* 33, no. 3: 543–554. https://doi.org/10.1111/j.1728-4457.2007.00184.x.

———. 2007b. "A New Perspective on Population Aging." *Demographic Research* 16 (January): 27–57. https://doi.org/10.4054/DemRes.2007.16.2.

———. 2008. "Conventional and Prospective Measures of Population Aging, 1995, 2005, 2025, 2045." Population Reference Bureau. http://www.prb.org/excel08/age-ageing_table.xls.

———. 2013. "The Characteristics Approach to the Measurement of Population Aging." *Population and Development Review* 39, no. 4: 673–685. https://doi.org/10.1111/j.1728-4457.2013.00633.x.

———. 2014. "Measuring the Speed of Aging across Population Subgroups." *PLoS ONE* 9, no. 5: e96289. https://doi.org/10.1371/journal.pone.0096289.

———. 2015a. "An Easily Understood and Intergenerationally Equitable Normal Pension Age." In *The Future of Welfare in a Global Europe,* edited by Bernd Marin, 193–220. Farnham, UK: Ashgate.

———. 2015b. "Are We Overly Dependent on Conventional Dependency Ratios?" *Population and Development Review* 41, no. 4: 687–708. https://doi.org/10.1111/j.1728-4457.2015.00091.x.

———. 2015c. "Faster Increases in Human Life Expectancy Could Lead to Slower Population Aging." *PLoS ONE* 10, no. 4: e0121922. https://doi.org/10.1371/journal.pone.0121922.

Sanderson, Warren C., Sergei Scherbov, and Patrick Gerland. 2017. "Probabilistic Population Aging." *PLoS ONE* 12, no. 6: e0179171. https://doi.org/10.1371/journal.pone.0179171.

Sanderson, Warren C., Sergei Scherbov, Daniela Weber, and Valeria Bordone. 2016. "Combined Measures of Upper and Lower Body Strength and Subgroup Differences in Subsequent Survival among the Older Population of England." *Journal of Aging and Health* 28, no. 7: 1178–1193. https://doi.org/10.1177/0898264316656515.

Scherbov, Sergei, Marija Mamolo, Michaela Potančoková, Tomas Sobotka, and Krystof Zeman. 2016. "European Demographic Data Sheet 2016." Vienna: Wittgenstein Centre. http://www.populationeurope.org/download/files/VID_DataSheet2016_printfile.pdf.

Shoven, John B. 2010. "New Age Thinking: Alternative Ways of Measuring Age, Their Relationship to Labor Force Participation, Government Policies and GDP." In *Research Findings in the Economics of Aging,* edited by David A. Wise, 17–36. Chicago: University of Chicago Press.

Shoven, John B., and Gopi Shah Goda. 2010. "Adjusting Government Policies for Age Inflation." In *Demography and the Economy,* edited by John B. Shoven, 143–162. Chicago: University of Chicago Press. http://www.nber.org/chapters/c8410.

Siegel, Jacob S. 1993. *A Generation of Change: A Profile of America's Older Population*. New York: Russell Sage Foundation.

Siegel, Jacob S., and Maria Davidson. 1984. "Demographic and Socioeconomic Aspects of Aging in the United States." *Current Population Reports* 43, series P-23. Washington, DC: US Government Printing Office.

Skirbekk, Vegard, Elke Loichinger, and Daniela Weber. 2012. "Variation in Cognitive Functioning as a Refined Approach to Comparing Aging across Countries." *Proceedings of the National Academy of Sciences* 109, no. 3: 770–774. https://doi.org/10.1073/pnas.1112173109.

Social Security. n.d. "Otto von Bismarck." Social Security History. Accessed February 11, 2019. https://www.ssa.gov/history/ottob.html.

Spring Discovery. n.d. "Spring Discovery." Accessed December 17, 2018. https://www.springdisc.com/#approac.

Statistics Canada. 2016. "Table 384-0038—Gross Domestic Product, Expenditure-Based, Provincial and Territorial, Annual (Dollars Unless Otherwise Noted)." Ottawa, ON: CANSIM. http://www5.statcan.gc.ca/cansim/a46?lang=eng&childId=3840038&CORId=3764&viewId=4.

Strange Wondrous. 2008. "Quotations by Lee Segall." http://strangewondrous.net/browse/author/s/segall+lee.

Sullivan, Daniel F. 1971. "A Single Index of Mortality and Morbidity." *HSMHA Health Reports* 86, no. 4: 347–354. https://doi.org/10.2307/4594169.

Swift, Jonathan. 1726. *Travels into Several Remote Nations of the World by Lemuel Gulliver*. London: Benjamin Motte.

Sydenstricker, Edgar, and Willford I. King. 1921. "The Classification of the Population According to Income." *Journal of Political Economy* 29: 571–594.

Taylor, Paul. 2009. "Growing Old in America: Expectations vs. Reality: Overview and Executive Summary." Washington, DC: Pew Research Center. http://www.pewsocialtrends.org/2009/06/29/growing-old-in-america-expectations-vs-reality/.

Thane, Patricia M. 2001. "Changing Paradigms of Aging and Being Older." In *Aging: Culture, Health, and Social Change*, edited by D. N. Weisstub, D. C. Thomasma, S. Gauthier, and G. F. Tomossy, 1–14. Dordrecht: Springer. https://doi.org/10.1007/978-94-017-0677-3_1.

Thompson, Warren S., and Pascal K. Whelpton. 1930. "A Nation of Elders in the Making." *American Mercury* 19: 385–397.

———. 1933. *Population Trends in the United States*. New York: McGraw-Hill.

Thomson Reuters. n.d. "Web of Science." Accessed November 2, 2017. https://webofknowledge.com/.

Triathlon Inspires. n.d. "Sister Madonna Buder 'the Iron Nun.'" Accessed November 8, 2017. http://www.triathloninspires.com/mbuderstory.html.

United Nations. 1983. *Vienna International Plan of Action on Aging*. New York: United Nations. http://www.un.org/es/globalissues/ageing/docs/vipaa.pdf.

———. 2015. *World Population Ageing 2015*. ST/ESA/SER.A/390. New York: Department of Economic and Social Affairs, Population Division. http://www.un.org/en/development/desa/population/publications/pdf/ageing/WPA2015_Report.pdf.

————. 2017a. *World Population Ageing 2017*. New York: Department of Economic and Social Affairs, Population Division. https://www.un.org/en/development/desa/population/publications/pdf/ageing/WPA2017_Report.pdf.

————. 2017b. *World Population Ageing 2017: Highlights*. New York: Department of Economic and Social Affairs, Population Division. http://www.un.org/en/development/desa/population/publications/pdf/ageing/WPA2017_Highlights.pdf.

————. 2017c. *World Population Prospects: The 2017 Revision*. New York: Department of Economic and Social Affairs, Population Division. https://population.un.org/wpp/.

————. 2017d. *World Population Prospects: The 2017 Revision. Classification of Countries by Region, Income Group and Subregion of the World*. New York: Department of Economic and Social Affairs, Population Division. https://esa.un.org/unpd/wpp/General/Files/Definition_of_Regions.pdf.

————. 2017e. *World Population Prospects: The 2017 Revision. Mortality Indicators*. New York: Department of Economic and Social Affairs, Population Division. https://population.un.org/wpp/Download/Standard/Mortality/.

————. 2017f. *World: Profiles of Ageing 2017*. New York: Department of Economic and Social Affairs, Population Division. https://population.un.org/ProfilesOfAgeing2017/index.html.

University of California, Berkeley. n.d. "United States Mortality Database." Accessed January 3, 2019. https://usa.mortality.org/.

University of California, Berkeley, and Max Planck Institute for Demographic Research. 2017. "Human Mortality Database." http://www.mortality.org.

Vaupel, James W. 2010. "Biodemography of Human Ageing." *Nature* 464: 536–542. https://doi.org/10.1038/nature08984.

VID (Vienna Institute of Demography of the Austrian Academy of Sciences) and IIASA (International Institute for Applied Systems Analysis). 2014. "European Demographic Datasheet 2014." Vienna: Wittgenstein Centre (IIASA, VID/OEAW, WU). https://www.oeaw.ac.at/en/vid/data/demographic-data-sheets/european-demographic-data-sheet-2014/.

————. 2016. "European Demographic Datasheet 2016." Vienna: Wittgenstein Centre (IIASA, VID/OEAW, WU). https://www.oeaw.ac.at/en/vid/about/news/details/article/european-demographic-data-sheet-2016/.

Weber, Daniela, Vegard Skirbekk, Inga Freund, and Agneta Herlitz. 2014. "The Changing Face of Cognitive Gender Differences in Europe." *Proceedings of the National Academy of Sciences* 111, no. 32: 11673–11678. https://doi.org/10.1073/pnas.1319538111.

Whelpton, Pascal K. 1932. "Increase and Distribution of Elders in Our Population." *Journal of the American Statistical Association* 27: 92–101. https://doi.org/10.2307/2277850

————. 1935. "Why the Large Rise in the German Birth-Rate?" *American Journal of Sociology* 41: 299–313.

WHO (World Health Organization). 2015. *World Report on Ageing and Health 2015*. Geneva, Switzerland: World Health Organization.

———. 2017a. "Child Growth Standards: Q. Will the Standards Be Applicable to All Children?" Geneva, Switzerland: World Health Organization. http://www.who.int/childgrowth/faqs/applicable/en/.

———. 2017b. "The WHO Child Growth Standards." Geneva, Switzerland: World Health Organization. http://www.who.int/childgrowth/standards/en/.

WHO and US National Institute on Aging. 2011. "Global Health and Aging." http://www.who.int/ageing/publications/global_health.pdf?ua=1.

Wikipedia. n.d.a. "Calico." Accessed November 2, 2017. https://en.wikipedia.org/wiki/Calico_(company).

———. n.d.b. "Madonna Buder." Accessed November 8, 2017. https://en.wikipedia.org/wiki/Madonna_Buder.

———. n.d.c. "Population Ageing." Accessed August 23, 2017. https://en.wikipedia.org/wiki/Population_ageing.

———. n.d.d. "Ufa." Accessed October 9, 2017. https://en.wikipedia.org/wiki/Ufa.

———. n.d.e. "Zlatoust." Accessed October 9, 2017. https://en.wikipedia.org/wiki/Zlatoust.

Wolford, Monica L., Kathleen Palso, and Anita Bercovitz. 2015. "Hospitalization for Total Hip Replacement among Inpatients Aged 45 and Over: United States, 2000–2010." In *NCHS Data Brief 186*. Hyattsville, MD: National Center for Health Statistics. https://www.cdc.gov/nchs/data/databriefs/db186.pdf.

Wong, Grace. 2016. "Northwestern Team Competes for $1M Prize to Slow Aging." *Chicago Tribune*, January 25, 2016. http://www.chicagotribune.com/business/ct-longevity-research-prize-northwestern-1126-biz-20160125-story.html.

World Association of Masters Athletes. n.d. "World Masters Athletics." Accessed November 8, 2017. https://www.world-masters-athletics.org/home.htm.

World Bank. 2016. "Live Long and Prosper: Aging in East Asia and Pacific." In *World Bank East Asia and Pacific Regional Report*. Washington, DC: World Bank. https://openknowledge.worldbank.org/bitstream/handle/10986/23133/9781464804694.pdf.

———. 2017. "World Bank Country and Lending Groups." Washington, DC: World Bank. https://datahelpdesk.worldbank.org/knowledgebase/articles/906519-world-bank-country-and-lending-groups.

Xu, Jiaquan, Sherry L. Murphy, Kenneth D. Kochanek, Brigham Bastian, and Elizabeth Arias. 2018. "Deaths: Final Data for 2016." National Vital Statistics Reports. Hyattsville, MD: National Center for Health Statistics. https://www.cdc.gov/nchs/data/nvsr/nvsr67/nvsr67_05.pdf.

ACKNOWLEDGMENTS

Behind each book is a story of its creation. Our story begins almost two decades ago and is set in a palace just south of Vienna, Austria. It is called Schloss Laxenburg (Laxenburg Palace), and it was originally built in the mid-1700s, when Maria Theresa was empress of Austria. The palace is now located on a beautiful public park that was once the private hunting grounds for Austrian aristocracy. It is the more recent of the two palaces on the grounds. The older one, many times renovated, was originally built in the mid-1300s. Our office is on the ground floor looking out at this beautiful park. In the upstairs/downstairs world of the aristocracy, our office is downstairs, perhaps where the servants used to perform their duties or where the children were cared for.

Our story is set here because of an agreement reached between NATO countries and Warsaw Pact countries to bring their scientists together in a neutral country to study problems of common concern. The organization where scientists continue to come together for that purpose is called the International Institute for Applied Systems Analysis (IIASA), and it remains in the palace. This book is one of the many fruits of that agreement.

At IIASA, we are currently members of the World Population Program, headed by Wolfgang Lutz. Lutz, through the dint of his hardwork, dedication to demography, and open and sharing personality, has managed to make the Vienna area one of the centers for demographic research in the world. The enthusiasm in the Vienna area for new thinking about demographic issues is one reason that the book was produced there.

The book was produced with support from the European Research Council under the European Union's Seventh Framework Programme (FP7 / 2007–2013) under grant agreement no. 323947.

There are many people who helped make this book what it is. Chief among these is Stefanie Andruchowitz. Her contributions have been so varied, so crucial, and so professionally performed that we do not know whether we could have completed the book without her. The book and many of its related research papers were supported by the EU grant. One of Ms. Andruchowitz's official duties was to administer the grant, and she did so with the utmost professionalism. Her contributions, however, went far beyond this. She also mastered the content of what we were writing. So, she was able to edit the book, not only for grammar and style, but also for substance. She has greatly improved it. We appreciate how unusual it is to find the skills of an administrator, editor, and consultant on substance all in one person.

Others also gave valuable comments. William Butz, Todd Goldman, Stanley Hale, Carol Sanderson, Mara Sanderson, and Annette Shidler provided helpful and detailed suggestions. Janice Audet of Harvard University Press provided advice about the style and organization of the book that were important for improving the consistency and the flow of ideas.

We would also like to thank the referees of the book. Their comments resulted in many additions, improvements, and clarifications.

Although the palace is the main setting for the story of this book, other important places played a role as well. Warren Sanderson was Professor of Economics at Stony Brook University while the book was being written, and his research on this book was supported there. Sergei Scherbov was part-time at the Vienna Institute of Demography (VID) and the Russian Presidential Academy of Economy and Public Administration (RANEPA). Both IIASA and the VID are partners in the Wittgenstein Centre for Demography and Global Human Capital (IIASA, VID/OEAW, WU), whose members provided a stimulating intellectual environment.

INDEX

f: Entry can be found in a figure.
t: Entry can be found in a table.

Academic literature: on age differences, 132; on onset of old age, 52–57, 59–60, 100

Activity limitations in old age, 115–127

Africa. *See also specific countries*: old-age dependency ratio and POADR in, 183, 184, 184*f*

Age differences and age difference trajectories, 128–167; and α-gender gaps in survival, 153–167, 233; definitions of, 13, 233; examples of, 129–132, 130*t*, 131*t*; female advantage in, 156–157; in Russian Federation, 13, 133–139, 140*f*–143*f*, 144–145; in standard population, 236; survey-based characteristics in, 94–95, 95*f*; in United States, 13, 133, 144–152, 146*f*–151*f*

Age distribution by country, UN data on, 7

Albania: median age and PMA in, 177*t*; old-age dependency ratio and POADR in, 174*t*

Alcohol consumption, 139, 145, 152

α-age of someone chronological age *x*, 96–99, 233

α-ages, 11, 85–87, 87*t*, 228; characteristics in, 11, 128–129; computation of, 96–99, 129; definition of, 233; difference between chronological age and (*See* Age differences and age difference trajectories); and life table characteristics, 91–94, 93*f*; and

prospective ages, 11, 235; in standard population, 96–99, 128–129, 233, 236

α-gender gaps in survival, 153–167; country comparisons of, 160–166, 161*t*–166*t*; definition of, 233; methodology in, 158–160, 167; in standard population, 236

Animal models: on gender gaps in survival and life expectancy, 154; on longevity, 169

Armenia: median age and PMA in, 173, 175*t*, 176, 177*t*; old-age dependency ratio and POADR in, 171, 172*t*, 173, 174*t*

Asia. *See also specific countries*: old-age dependency ratio and POADR in, 183, 184, 185*f*, 190, 191*f*–193*f*

Athletic accomplishments in old age, 49–50

Australia: age differences in, 159*t*, 159–160; α-ages in, 93*f*; α-gender gaps in survival in, 160–162, 161*t*, 163*t*, 163–164; constant characteristic ages in, 91, 92*f*; Daw's measure of female advantage in, 157; prospective ages of 65-year olds in, 40*t*, 41

Austria: economic support ratio in, 81; median age and PMA in, 177*t*; old-age dependency ratio and POADR in, 174*t*; prospective ages of 65-year olds in, 40*t*, 41; prospective old-age thresholds in, 119*t*, 121*t*, 123*t*–125*t*; self-reporting of health